Sexual Heal[th] and Genital Medicine

WC 140 SON

50149
£5.00

D1642786

MEDICAL AND PROFESSIONAL LIBRARY
DONCASTER ROYAL INFIRMARY
TEL: 642894

DRI LIBRARY SERVICE
WITHDRAWN
FROM STOCK

23. DEC 2008

13 OCT 2014

This book should be returned by the last date stamped above. You may renew the loan for a further period if the book is not required by another reader.

26 APR 2007

Sexual Health and Genital Medicine in Clinical Practice

Chris Sonnex

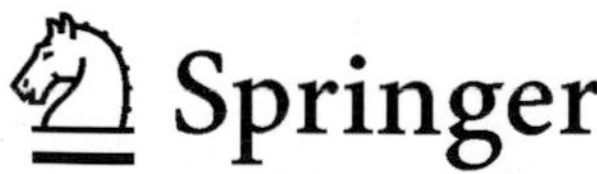

PROPERTY OF DONCASTER ROYAL INFIRMARY LIBRARY

Dr Chris Sonnex FRCP
Department of GenitoUrinary Medicine,
Addenbrooke's Hospital, Cambridge University Hospitals NHS Foundation Trust, Cambridge, UK

British Library Cataloguing in Publication Data
A catalogue record for this book is available from the British Library

Library of Congress Control Number: 2006934989

ISBN-10: 1-84628-406-6 e-ISBN-10: 1-84628-416-3
ISBN-13: 978-1-84628-406-9 e-ISBN-13: 978-1-84628-416-8

Printed on acid-free paper.

© Springer-Verlag London Limited 2007

Apart from any fair dealing for the purposes of research or private study, or criticism or review, as permitted under the Copyright, Designs and Patents Act of 1988, this publication may only be reproduced, stored or transmitted, in any form or by any means, with the prior permission in writing of the publishers, or in the case of reprographic reproduction in accordance with the terms of licences issued by the Copyright Licensing Agency. Enquiries concerning reproduction outside those terms should be sent to the publishers.

The use of registered names, trademarks, etc. in this publication does not imply, even in the absence of a specific statement, that such names are exempt from the relevant laws and regulations and therefore free for general use.

Product liability: The publisher can give no guarantee for information about drug dosage and application thereof contained in this book. In every individual case the respective user must check its accuracy by consulting other pharmaceutical literature.

9 8 7 6 5 4 3 2 1

Springer Science+Business Media
springer.com

Contents

Preface

This book is aimed specifically at medical practitioners in primary care who require a quick guide to help diagnose and manage genital problems. As such this is not a comprehensive text but a prompt to "what to do next" when faced with a patient presenting with a genital complaint. A list of reference textbooks is provided in Further Reading and I would suggest you have at least one of these available for perusing at a more leisurely pace at a later time.

Just a word of explanation about "Genitourinary Medicine", which is referred to in the text and is familiar to practitioners in the United Kingdom. "GU medicine" arose as a medical specialty in the mid-1980s replacing the term "Venereology" which seemed an outdated and too restrictive description for the types of problems seen in, the then, so-called "VD" or "special" clinics. Although many patients attended these clinics with sexually transmitted infections (STIs), a good number attended with other genital problems. GU medicine clinicians now routinely diagnose and manage genital skin conditions, psychosexual problems, and infections, such as candidiasis and bacterial vaginosis, in addition to sexually acquired infections. The name "genitourinary medicine" was considered more appropriate and less stigmatizing as it suggests a specialty that deals with a range of medical conditions affecting the urogenital tract. "GU medicine" has caused some confusion beyond the UK, but education rather than reverting back to old title of "STI clinician" is the preferred way forward. The stigma associated with STIs persists and, inevitably, a degree of stigma hangs over the GU medicine clinic, but the message that GU medicine has a wider sexual health remit is slowly permeating through the medical establishment and into the public psyche. Over the last few years in the UK, there has been a trend to move away from the name "GU medicine" toward "sexual health". This is by no means favored by all and does lead to a blurring of the remit of the specialty and some loss of identity, as gynecologists and family planning specialists would also, quite rightly, consider their expertise to fall within the umbrella term "sexual health". Training will eventually provide expertise in all aspects of sexual health care but for the moment, in the UK at least, GU medicine has a well-defined training program with the emphasis on genital infection and STI diagnosis and management.

This text attempts to cover the range of conditions seen in GU medicine clinics in the UK but genital infections and medical problems are pretty similar worldwide and so any practitioner managing genital disease and sexual health problems should find this book of practical value.

Chapter 1

Which Patients to Refer to Genitourinary Medicine

There is an appreciable overlap between genitourinary (GU) medicine and gynecology, urology and dermatology, which sometimes leads to difficulties when deciding to whom to turn for further advice or a specialist opinion. The following should be considered as general guidelines: if in doubt to whom to refer, give your local GU medicine clinic a call.

Many consultants in GU medicine have specific interests and the services available from individual clinics may vary accordingly. A large number of clinics provide expertise in vulval disease, genital dermatology, psychosexual medicine, colposcopy, and sexual assault assessment and management. Getting to know your local department of GU medicine or sexual health is to be strongly recommended: GU medicine clinicians are usually very approachable and are delighted to have general practitioners (GPs) and practice nurses attend clinical sessions and learn more about the specialty.

1.1 CONSIDER URGENT REFERRAL

Men with

- Urethral discharge or dysuria
- Acute epididymitis.

Men and women with

- Primary genital herpes
- Genital ulceration: Previously unconfirmed diagnosis.

1.2 REFERRAL STRONGLY RECOMMENDED

Men and women with

- Concern (patient or doctor) regarding sexually transmitted infection

- Concern regarding human immunodeficiency virus (HIV) infection
- Any of the following infections (proven or suspected):
  - chlamydial infection
  - non-gonococcal urethritis
  - gonorrhea
  - trichomoniasis.
- Sexual partners of patients with
  - chlamydial infection
  - non-gonococcal urethritis
  - gonorrhea
  - trichomoniasis.
- Positive syphilis serology.

1.3 REFERRAL RECOMMENDED

Women with

- Persistent/recurrent vaginal discharge
- Persistent/recurrent vulval irritation/soreness/burning
- Chronic pelvic pain
- Dysuria/frequency with sterile urine culture.
- Young women with post-coital bleeding (possibly prior to referral to gynecology)
- Painful sexual intercourse (superficial or deep).

Men with

- "Testicular"/intrascrotal discomfort
- Symptoms suggestive of prostatitis/chronic pelvic pain syndrome
- Balanoposthitis.

Men and women with

- Genital warts
- Genital molluscum contagiosum
- Genital "lumps" of uncertain etiology
- Pubic lice
- Genital rashes (diagnosis uncertain or unresponsive to treatment).

1.4 CONSIDER REFERRAL

Women with recurrent candidiasis or recurrent bacterial vaginosis.

Chapter 2
Routine Investigations Performed in Genitourinary Medicine

Patients attending a GU medicine department for the first time and those presenting with new problems will usually undergo a variety of investigations to check for evidence of infection, both sexually and non-sexually acquired. Many GPs are uncertain which tests are routinely performed and a standard letter from the clinic stating that "the screen for genital infection proved negative" is not particularly instructive. All clinics should be screening for the same infections; however, the specific tests used may vary from clinic to clinic.

Tests routinely performed are as follows.

2.1 MEN

2.1.1 Urethral Swab

- *Gram stain – microscopy
  >4 polymorphs per high power field (HPF) = urethritis
  Gram-negative diplococci within polymorphs – *presumptive* diagnosis of gonococcal urethritis
- Culture for *Neisseria gonorrhoeae* (definitive diagnosis of gonorrhea).
- *Chlamydia trachomatis* detection (usually by nucleic acid amplification test (NAAT) (e.g. PCR or LCR) or enzyme immunoassay (EIA)).

Some clinics have now moved from urethral swab to urine testing for *Chlamydia* detection. This is likely to become the favored method (certainly by patients) for diagnosing urethral chlamydial infection in men.

2.1.2 *Two Glass Urine Test

This is a time-honored test performed in UK GU medicine clinics, considered by some to be of debatable value. It certainly can help to differentiate a pure urethritis (usually sexually acquired) from a urethritis in association with a cystitis (i.e. a UTI, and not sexually acquired).

- First glass = a first catch urine (50 ml)
- Second glass = second part of urinary stream (50 ml)

Any remaining urine is passed into the urinal.
The following are the interpretation of urine results:

(1) First: clear; second: clear = normal
(2) First: pus (seen as threads, flakes, general haze); second: clear = anterior urethritis (e.g. non-gonococcal urethritis (NGU), gonorrhea)
(3) First: pus; second: pus = posterior urethritis or cystitis (e.g. *E. coli*, etc.). Send the first glass urine or mid-stream urine (MSU) for culture.

Phosphaturia is a common cause of cloudy urine. The addition of acetic acid will clear the urine when excess phosphates are present whereas the haze remains in cases of pyuria.

The urine may also be checked by dipstix.

Some UK clinics no longer look for urethritis in asymptomatic men. There is however concern that cases of *Mycoplasma genitalium* urethritis may be missed as culture and nucleic acid amplification tests are not currently routinely available for diagnosing this infection.

The details for women are summarized in Table 2.1.

2.2 MEN AND WOMEN

2.2.1 Syphilis Serology

A blood sample is routinely taken for syphilis serology. There are a number of serological tests available for diagnosing syphilis; commonly used ones include *Treponema pallidum* antibody, VDRL, and TPHA or TPPA. Screening in GU medicine and antenatal clinics and on donating blood for transfusion has proved

*Indicates tests that may not be currently available or performed in all clinics.

TABLE 2.1. Routine tests performed on women.

Procedure	Test	Diagnosis
*Vaginal swab	Gram stain: microscopy	Assess bacterial flora Bacterial vaginosis Candidiasis
	Wet mount: microscopy	Trichomoniasis Candidiasis
	Culture	*Candida* *Trichomonas vaginalis*
Cervical swab	*Gram stain: microscopy	>30 polymorphs/HPF suggests cervicitis Gram-negative diplococci inside polymorphs → presumptive diagnosis of gonorrhea
	Culture	*Neisseria gonorrhoeae*
Cervical swab	*Chlamydia trachomatis* detection (e.g. EIA, NAAT)	
Cervical cytology	(if indicated)	
*Urethral swab	Gram stain: microscopy	Polymorphs may be seen in: chlamydial infection, gonorrhea, trichomoniasis. Gram-negative diplococci inside polymorphs → presumptive diagnosis of gonorrhea
	Culture	*Neisseria gonorrhoeae*
Urethral swab	*Chlamydia trachomatis* detection (e.g. EIA, NAAT)	

*many clinics no longer perform microscopic assessment of vaginal and cervical samples in asymptomatic women and who are not contacts of a partner with an STI.

successful in keeping syphilis prevalence extremely low in the UK, although in very recent years we have seen an increase in syphilis prevalence in certain areas.

2.2.2 Hepatitis Screening

Many clinics offer hepatitis B screening and vaccination for injecting drug users and homosexual men and hepatitis C screening for injecting drug users.

2.2.3 HIV Antibody Testing

This is now routinely offered to patients attending GU medicine clinics for screening or testing for STIs and to all women as part of their antenatal care in England and Wales. Some clinics provide a "fast testing service" where results are available "while you wait" or the next day. This aims to encourage individuals to be tested who are otherwise deterred by the prospect of a wait for several days for the results.

Chapter 3
Taking a Sexual History

Whereas most patients attending GU medicine will expect to be asked questions about sex, this is by no means always the case in primary care, even though the patient may have presented with genital symptoms. GU medicine clinicians spend their days asking patients fairly intimate questions about sexual habits and lifestyle and therefore feel comfortable with the questions and the replies. Most GPs will only infrequently need to take a sexual history and a degree of uncertainty regarding which questions to ask and how best to ask them is inevitable. The purpose of this short chapter is to provide basic guidelines on how to approach the patient presenting with genital symptoms or who is concerned that they may have acquired an infection from a sexual partner.

An unmarried female patient presenting with vaginal discharge provides a useful example of one possible approach to sexual history taking.

The following are the important questions:

- How long has the discharge been present?
- Is there any malodor (? bacterial vaginosis)
  - Is there any associated vulval irritation or soreness (? candidiasis)
  - Is the discharge white (? candidiasis, bacterial vaginosis) or yellow (? trichomoniasis, cervicitis)
- Have there ever been any previous similar episodes? If so:
  - What was the diagnosis?
  - Which treatments have been used?
  - Have any previous treatments helped?
- Have you experienced any pelvic pain (? endometritis/pelvic inflammatory disease (PID))
- Has there been any bleeding between periods? (endometritis)
- When was your last period?
- Has there been any discomfort or pain during sexual intercourse? (the terms "when making love" or "when having sex"

are preferred by some clinicians; use whichever you think will be appropriate for the patient and with which you feel comfortable)

- When did you last have intercourse/have sex/make love?
- Was it your regular partner?
  (1) If no:
    - Was it with someone you know well or a fairly casual contact (? able to contact again)?
    - Was it a male partner or a female partner?
    - Was he or she from this country?
    - Had they recently spent any time abroad?
    - Have you had sex with any other partners in the past few months?

  (2) If yes:
    - Is this a male partner or a female partner?
    - When did you last have sexual contact with someone other than your regular partner? (This may be more appropriate left to the end of the consultation.)
      Direct eye-to-eye contact usually works best for the more intimate questions. The last question can be difficult as patients are usually embarrassed to admit an "extramarital" or casual affair, so you need to try to achieve a lack of surprise and concern whatever the reply.
    - If a male partner, has he mentioned that he has symptoms? For example, a penile rash or any discomfort passing urine?
    - What are you using for contraception? (consistent use of condoms provides good protection against *Chlamydia* and gonorrhea)
    - Are you currently on any medication? (some antibiotics predispose to candidiasis. Fixed drug eruptions may present as fairly extensive areas of erythema or ulceration on the external genitalia.)

You will appreciate that a number of these questions are aimed specifically at determining the risk of sexually transmitted infection. They may not be relevant to the patient with clinically obvious vaginal "thrush" but should be considered in women with, for example, troublesome vaginal discharge unresponsive to treatment.

If a woman's last sexual contact was with another woman, it is worth enquiring when they last had sexual contact with a man. Women who are exclusively lesbian are unlikely to have chlamydial or gonococcal infection whereas bacterial vaginosis appears to be slightly more common in lesbian than in heterosexual women.

A similar line of questioning to the above is required for men attending with genital symptoms such as dysuria, urethral discharge, epididymal tenderness, or genital ulceration. You should directly inquire the following:

- When they last had sexual intercourse
- Whether it was with a "regular" or "casual" partner
- Whether it was with a male or female partner
- Whether there have been other sexual contacts in the previous few months.

With men who have sex with men (MSM), one should also obtain a little more detail about clinically relevant sexual practices. For example:

- Do you usually practice "safe-sex"? (e.g. body-rubbing, mutual masturbation)?
- When did you last have penetrative intercourse?
- When you have penetrative intercourse do you usually penetrate your partner (ano-insertive) or does he penetrate you (ano-receptive) or is there both?
  - if predominantly ano-insertive, when were you last ano-receptive?
  - if predominantly ano-receptive, when were you last ano-insertive?
  - do you routinely/always use condoms?
  - are you having any problems with condoms splitting or tearing? (extra strong condoms are readily available; certain lubricants can damage condom latex (see 'Condoms', Chapter 12)
- When did you last have oral sex? (Some infections can be passed from the throat to the urethra, e.g. non-specific urethritis (NSU), gonorrhea. HIV may also be transmitted by oro-genital contact.)
- Were you active and/or receptive? (i.e. your penis into partner's mouth or vice versa).

Other sexual practices that may lead to the transmission of infection or clinical complications include the following:

- "Rimming" (oro-anal contact): intestinal pathogens, hepatitis A
- "Fisting" (hand insertion into rectum): damage to the anal sphincter, rectal tears.

The issue of HIV infection should be raised if the history suggests a possibility of potentially risky sexual practices. Recent studies suggest that a number of young homosexual men perceive HIV as a problem affecting the "older generation" and are reverting to unsafe sexual practices, in particular unprotected anal intercourse with casual partners.

Syphilis is also appearing once again in the UK with oral sex proving an important route of spread amongst men who have sex with men.

Chapter 4
Bacterial Vaginosis

Bacterial vaginosis (BV) is more common than "thrush" and is probably the commonest cause of abnormal vaginal discharge seen in primary care. The condition is certainly underdiagnosed and frequently misdiagnosed. BV was formerly known as "Gardnerella" and is caused by an overgrowth of predominantly anaerobic bacterial species which are commonly present in low concentrations in a healthy vagina (e.g. *Gardnerella vaginalis*, *Prevotella* spp., *Peptostreptococcus*, *Mobiluncus*, *Mycoplasma hominis*).

Although many clinicians regard BV as a fairly insignificant condition, this is certainly not the case for the majority of sufferers. Many women find the amount of discharge, and in some cases the associated malodor, to be particularly distressing. In addition, there is increasing evidence that BV is associated with preterm labor, late miscarriage, chorioamnionitis, postpartum endometritis and bacteremia, pelvic infection following surgery and termination of pregnancy, and, possibly, PID.

4.1 SYMPTOMS

The commonest presenting symptom is excessive vaginal discharge, sometimes with a slight malodor. Some women regard a fishy vaginal odor as normal and are surprised and grateful when BV is eventually diagnosed and treated. Malodor may only be noticeable after unprotected sexual intercourse, owing to the release of amines by alkaline semen (see "Amine test" below). Vulval irritation is uncommon. As with candidiasis, many women with BV are asymptomatic.

4.2 DIAGNOSIS

The following are the two most important methods of diagnosis.

(1) Microscopy of vaginal secretions
BV produces a highly characteristic appearance on Gram staining. There is an absence of lactobacilli and an excess of

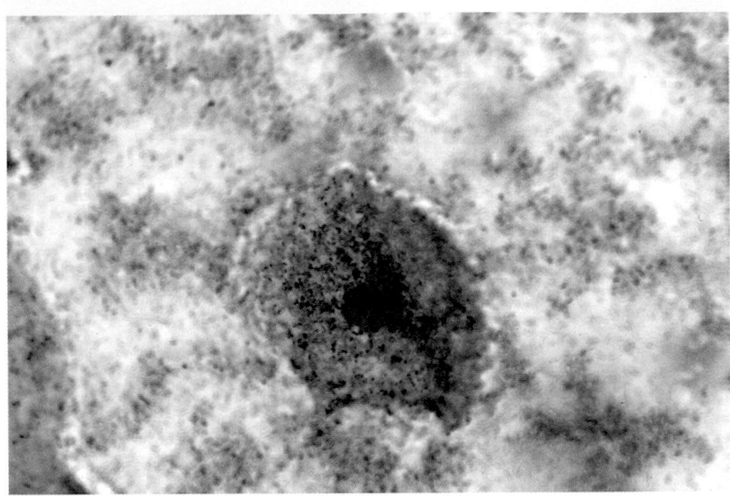

FIGURE 4.1. Gram stain of vaginal discharge due to bacterial vaginosis – lactobacilli replaced by *Gardnerella vaginalis, Prevotella* species, *Mycoplasma hominis,* peptostreptococci and other predominantly anaerobic bacteria

Gram-variable or Gram-negative rods (*Gardnerella, Prevotella, Peptostreptococcus*; Figures 4.1 and 4.2). In some cases Gram-negative "curved rods" (*Mobiluncus*) may be seen. As vaginal inflammation (vaginitis) is not a feature of BV, few polymorphs are present.

(2) Amine test

This test involves the addition of two drops of 1–5% potassium hydroxide solution to a sample of the vaginal secretions, either on a slide or on a swab. The sudden release of a fishy odor represents a "positive" result. The odor results from volatilization of polyamines, in particular trimethylamine, that are thought to be produced by the anaerobic bacteria.

Compared with microscopy, the "amine test" has a sensitivity of 80–90% and a specificity of well over 90%. The test is easy, quick, and inexpensive to perform and should be part of the initial assessment of all women with vaginal discharge.

Although the amine test may be performed on air-dried swabs some hours or days later, the main advantage of the test is that it can be performed during the consultation. The odor produced is short lasting and, despite some claims to the contrary, does not linger in the room where the test is performed. Testing is probably best performed out of sight of the patient.

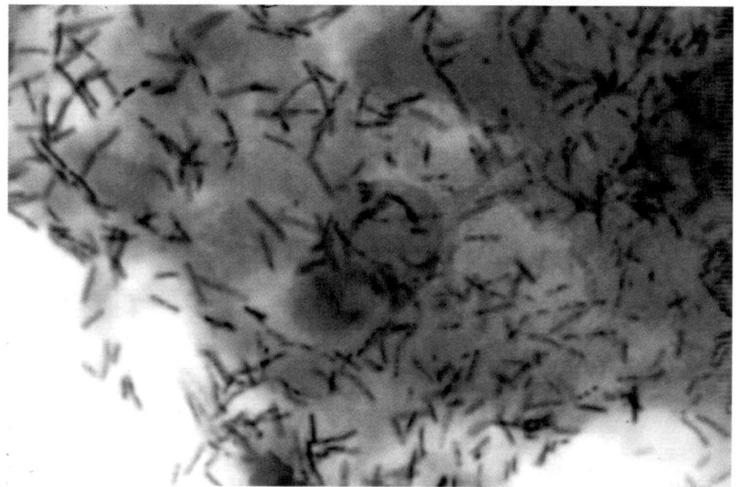

FIGURE 4.2. Gram stain of vaginal secretions showing lactobacilli

The following are other diagnostic criteria mentioned in the textbooks but less helpful than microscopy and amine testing.

(3) Vaginal pH
In BV, vaginal pH is raised from the normal value of 4.5 to above 5.0. Unfortunately, this is not specific and probably signifies simply a reduction in the number of lactobacilli. (Lactobacilli are the predominant bacterial species in the healthy vagina and maintain a protective acid environment in the vagina by, we think, producing lactic acid from vaginal glycogen.) In addition, a raised pH may be found in a woman with a normal vaginal flora if testing is performed when menstrual blood or semen is present or if cervical mucus is inadvertently sampled instead of vaginal secretions. BV, however, is very unlikely to be present if the pH is normal.

(4) Appearance of the discharge
Although the vaginal discharge in BV is classically thin, homogeneous with a creamy or milky consistency and a slight froth (Figure. 4.3), this is by no means always the case, and in most studies the appearance of vaginal fluid has been shown to be a poor diagnostic marker.

High vaginal swab culture has no place in diagnosis because the presence of *Gardnerella vaginalis* or anaerobes does not necessarily indicate the presence of bacterial

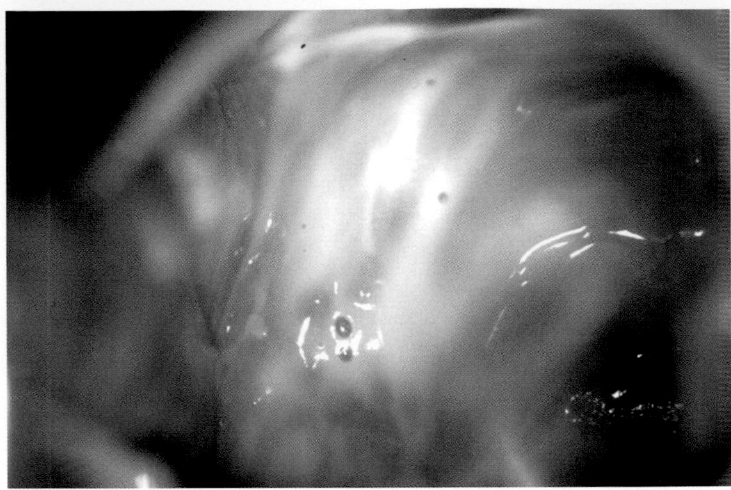

FIGURE 4.3. Bacterial vaginosis – creamy, homogeneous discharge coating the vaginal wall

vaginosis. Quantitative culture may be helpful but it is difficult to perform. As mentioned above, microscopy is the diagnostic test of choice.

4.3 TREATMENT

There are a few options available.

- Oral metronidazole is an extremely effective treatment and various regimens have been used: 2 g suspension stat dose; 400–500 mg bd for 5 days; 200 mg tds for 7 days.
- Intravaginal metronidazole gel (0.75%) daily for 5 days.

Patients should be advised to avoid alcohol whilst taking metronidazole (possibly also when used intravaginally) owing to a disulfiram effect.

- Intravaginal clindamycin cream (2%) daily for seven days is a useful alternative for patients who cannot tolerate metronidazole (worth mentioning to patient that clindamycin cream may weaken condoms).
- Oral clindamycin 300 mg bd for 7 days.

Treatment is currently reserved for women with symptoms. A case could be made for treating asymptomatic women prior to hysterectomy, endometrial biopsy, termination of pregnancy, dilatation and curettage (D & C), and intrauterine contraceptive device (IUCD) insertion, although there are no studies supporting this for the latter two procedures. The possibility of inoculating the uterus with bacteria capable of causing endometrial infection does lend support to the suggestion that BV should be treated prior to any procedure involving instrumentation through the cervix.

Trials are ongoing to assess whether treating BV in pregnancy reduces the risk of preterm labor. Studies performed to date have given conflicting results; however, some of those failing to show a benefit have been criticized regarding the timing of diagnosis. Diagnosing and treating BV very early in pregnancy may be important. It is reasonable to say that on current evidence treatment should be considered in pregnant women with a past history of preterm labor of uncertain cause or late miscarriage, and that treatment should be given as early as possible in the pregnancy. The drugs recommended for treating BV are safe to use in pregnancy. Meta-analyses show no evidence of teratogenicity with metronidazole.

4.4 RECURRENT BACTERIAL VAGINOSIS

A recurrence is seen in about 20% of women after treatment irrespective of the drug used. This is often a "bacteriological" recurrence (i.e. BV is diagnosed on microscopy) rather than symptomatic recurrence. However, some women do experience frequent symptomatic recurrences which, as with recurrent candidiasis, often affect sexual relationships and cause a degree of psychological morbidity. Treating sexual partners has been shown to have no effect on reducing the recurrence rate. There is an association between BV and the IUCD and in women with particularly troublesome recurrences an alternative form of contraception should be considered. Using condoms for a few months may prove beneficial for some patients.

A short course (2–3 days) of oral metronidazole or intravaginal clindamycin or metronidazole once or twice a month may also be worth considering as a prophylactic measure (the necessary studies are awaited). In addition, recent reports have suggested benefit from using an intravaginal acid gel after standard treatment with metronidazole.

Chapter 5
Candidiasis

General practitioners are all too familiar with this condition, so there is little to be gained by reiterating common knowledge. There are, however, a few points worth making.

Although *C. albicans* is the commonest cause of vulvovaginal infection, other strains such as *Candida* (formerly *Torulopsis*) *glabrata* and *Candida tropicalis*, may also occasionally produce symptoms. *C. glabrata* is thought to account for about 5% of vaginal infections.

Accurate identification of *Candida* spp. is particularly important when dealing with persistent or recurrent infection; however, this identification may not be available routinely in all microbiology laboratories. Non-*albicans* strains of *Candida* often show partial or complete resistance to the commonly used topical and oral antifungal agents.

Oral antifungals (e.g. fluconazole, itraconazole) are extremely effective, easy to use and appear to be safe. They are, however, rather more expensive than topical treatments and should not be used in pregnancy.

5.1 RECURRENT CANDIDIASIS

A small number of women are plagued by frequent recurrences of vulvovaginal candidiasis. The reasons are unclear, although there is some evidence to suggest a localized *Candida*-specific defect in cell-mediated immunity. When a patient presents complaining of "recurrent thrush," one of the most important first steps in management is to make sure that the diagnosis is correct (see below).

5.1.1 Practical Points

Whenever possible try to send a vaginal swab for *Candida* culture on each occasion that symptoms are present. Failure to culture the yeast makes the diagnosis less likely.

If symptoms persist and *Candida* continues to be isolated after treatment, ask the laboratory to identify the *Candida* species and report on its sensitivities to the various antifungals. This will usually require the sample being sent to a reference laboratory. Non-*albicans* strains of *Candida* are often resistant to imidazoles (e.g. clotrimazole, miconazole, econazole) and triazoles (fluconazole, itraconazole) but may respond to topical nystatin (a polyene).

Consider a trial of an oral antifungal, such as fluconazole 150 mg stat followed by 50 mg daily for 1 week or itraconazole 200 mg bd for 1 day followed by 200 mg daily for 1 week. Lack of clinical response suggests that *Candida* is not the cause of the symptoms or that a resistant strain of *Candida* is present. Symptoms of vulval irritation, with or without discharge, which initially improve with antifungal treatment but then recur some days or weeks later are highly suggestive of candidiasis.

5.2 DIFFERENTIAL DIAGNOSES

5.2.1 Bacterial Vaginosis

Consider **bacterial vaginosis** in a woman with recurrent vaginal discharge that fails to respond to antifungal treatment. Vulval irritation is unusual in this condition.

5.2.2 Vulal Dermatoses (see Chapter 8)

A reasonable number of women with presumed persistent (rather than recurrent) "thrush" have been misdiagnosed and have a dermatosis. Vulval seborrheic dermatitis, lichen sclerosus, and lichen planus are not uncommon but any skin condition can affect the genitalia. Dermatoses often lose some of their characteristic features when affecting the vulval epithelium and a biopsy may be required to make the correct diagnosis. Some patients with a vulval dermatosis will have other body sites affected. In cases of contact dermatitis, there is often a history of allergy or a family history of atopy. Potential vulval sensitizing agents include topical medications (e.g. Tri-adcortyl, antifungal creams), KY jelly (propylene glycol sensitivity), spermicidal creams, sanitary pads, dyed lavatory paper, bubble-baths, and scented soaps (although prolonged soaking in a bath rather than fleeting contact with showering is required to produce a hypersensitivity reaction).

5.3 MANAGEMENT OF RECURRENT CANDIDIASIS

Once you are satisfied that the diagnosis is correct the following points are worth considering.

5.3.1 Prophylactic Antifungals

Women with peri-menstrual thrush may benefit from prophylactic antifungal therapy either before or just after the period. This can be as a single clotrimazole 500 mg pessary or fenticonazole 600 mg pessary, oral fluconazole 150 mg or itraconazole 200 mg bd for 1 day. Once monthly prophylaxis is insufficient for some women in which case try fortnightly or possibly weekly prophylaxis. This regimen should be continued for 3-6 months and then stopped and the situation reassessed.

5.3.2 Treatment of Male Sexual Partners

Treating the male partner with an antifungal cream does not reduce the frequency of recurrent episodes in the female. Men should therefore only receive treatment if they have evidence of candidal infection themselves (i.e. a balanitis or posthitis).

5.3.3 Treatment of the "Gut Reservoir"

Early studies suggested that recurrences of vaginal candidiasis result from reinfection from the gut. This is now considered unlikely and indeed more recent work has failed to show any benefit from the use of oral nystatin. Intestinal colonization by *Candida* therefore appears to play no role in recurrent vaginal infection and can be ignored.

5.3.4 "Deep-Seated" Vaginal Infection

Failure to eradicate *Candida* from the "deeper layers" of the vaginal mucosa has led some clinicians to suggest using longer courses of antifungal treatment. This is still an issue of debate, but consider treating acute recurrences with a 2-week course of antifungal pessaries or oral agents.

5.3.5 Diet

There is no evidence to suggest that a diet high in sugars or carbohydrates predisposes to thrush. One study of particular interest reported a reduction in vaginal *Candida* colonization among women ingesting 8 ounces of yoghurt daily. A "natural" yoghurt was used, supposedly containing *Lactobacillus acidophilus*. Although this work still requires confirmation with a larger number of patients and a placebo arm, yoghurt supplementation sounds attractive and would probably be well accepted. Interestingly, many of the so-called "live" or "natural" yoghurt products on the market do not contain *Lactobacillus acidophilus* or contain only "non-vaginal" strains of lactobacilli. A small number of studies have shown an association between low zinc status and recurrent vaginal infection including recurrent candidiasis. This has led some clinicians to suggest a trial of oral zinc supplements for 1 or 2 months in women with particularly troublesome thrush. Garlic contains an antifungal, allicin, and has been advocated as a treatment for thrush; however, current evidence suggests that the amount of garlic required to provide clinically useful levels of allicin in the vagina may be socially unacceptable. Nevertheless, natural remedies are very fashionable and further study is certainly warranted.

5.3.6 Diabetes

Poorly controlled diabetes may predispose to thrush, but it is very uncommon to find diabetes in women with recurrent infection; however, it is prudent to dipstix the urine.

5.3.7 Oral Contraceptive Pill

Theoretical evidence suggests that the pill could play a role in potentiating vaginal candidiasis. A cytosol receptor for estrogen has been reported in *C. albicans* and certain hormones have been shown in vitro to stimulate yeast mycelial formation and hence virulence. In spite of this evidence, recent studies have failed to show an association between low-moderate dose oral contraceptive pill use and recurrent candidiasis.

5.3.8 Iron Deficiency Anemia

This does not predispose to recurrent thrush.

5.3.9 Bubble-Baths and Scented Soaps

The irritation associated with candidal vulvitis may be aggravated by bubble-baths and scented soaps. Conversely, epithelial damage due to a mild contact dermatitis to one of the chemicals in a bubble-bath or soap may predispose to symptomatic candidiasis.

5.3.10 Tight-Fitting Clothing

Women with recurrent thrush are often advised to avoid wearing nylon underwear and tights. The theory is that the increased humidity generated by the nylon may lead to mild epithelial maceration and subsequently lead to fungal invasion of the superficial tissue and hence to symptomatic infection. This is anecdotal but loose clothing does provide a degree of comfort to some women during recurrences.

5.3.11 Antibiotics

A number of women are prone to develop thrush during courses of oral antibiotics. This may be due to the elimination of the protective vaginal lactobacilli or to a direct potentiating effect on yeast growth. Prescribing a course of antifungals together with antibiotics is worth considering and is usually much appreciated by the patient.

5.3.12 Douches

Vinegar or sodium bicarbonate douches provide symptomatic relief for some women. It should be remembered that douching may facilitate the spread of lower genital tract bacteria into the uterus and is not to be generally recommended unless a screen for genital infection has been performed and proved negative.

5.3.13 Boric Acid

Gelatin capsules of boric acid have been successfully used to treat persistent vaginal candidiasis, in particular *C. glabrata* infection. The recommended dosage is 600 mg bd for two weeks and as the capsules are not generally available these need to be made up by a kindly pharmacist. As prolonged absorption of boric acid causes anorexia, vomiting, skin rash, and anemia, further study is required on the safety and efficacy of maintenance therapy.

5.3.14 Hormonal Therapy

There are anecdotal reports of successful treatments of persistent *C. glabrata* infection with progestogens, for example dydrogesterone or medroxyprogesterone acetate.

Summary of recurrent/persistent vaginal candidiasis

(1) Make sure that the diagnosis is correct. Dermatoses often present with vulval irritation.
(2) Identify the *Candida* spp. and check sensitivities to antifungals.
(3) Treat initially with a longer course of antifungals.
(4) Use monthly, fortnightly, or weekly oral or topical antifungals for 3–6 months as prophylaxis.
(5) No need to treat male partners with antifungals unless symptomatic (i.e. penile rash present).

The clinical and microscopic features of candidiasis are shown below (Figures 5.1–5.6). See also chapter 16 for candidiasis in men.

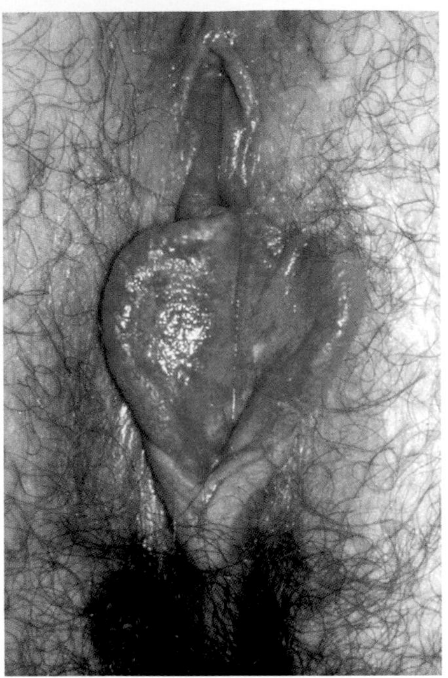

FIGURE 5.1(a). Vulvitis due to candidiasis

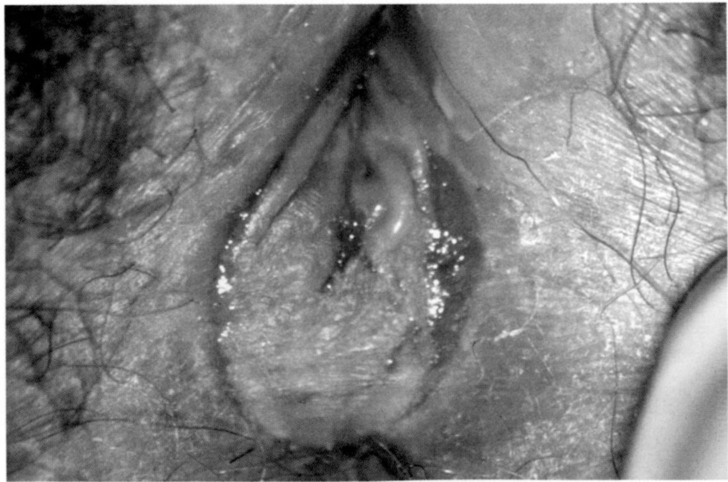

FIGURE 5.1(b). Perineal fissures due to candidiasis

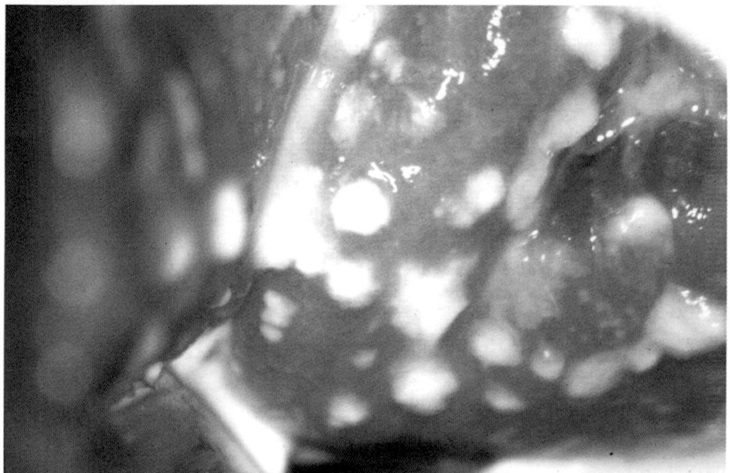

FIGURE 5.2. Candidiasis – 'lumpy' white discharge

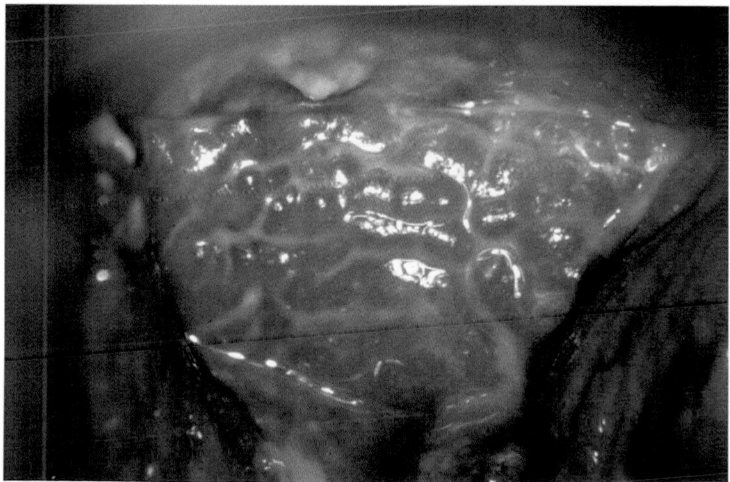

FIGURE 5.3. Candidiasis – vaginitis with a watery discharge

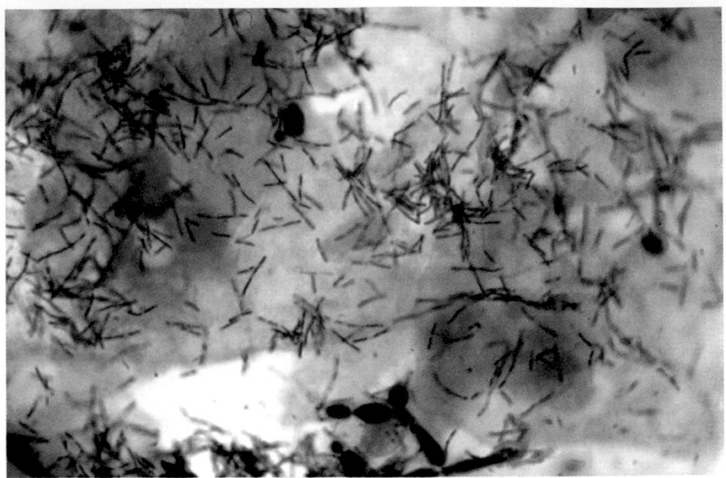

FIGURE 5.4. Gram stain of vaginal discharge due to candidiasis showing spores and pseudo-hyphae (lactobacilli also present)

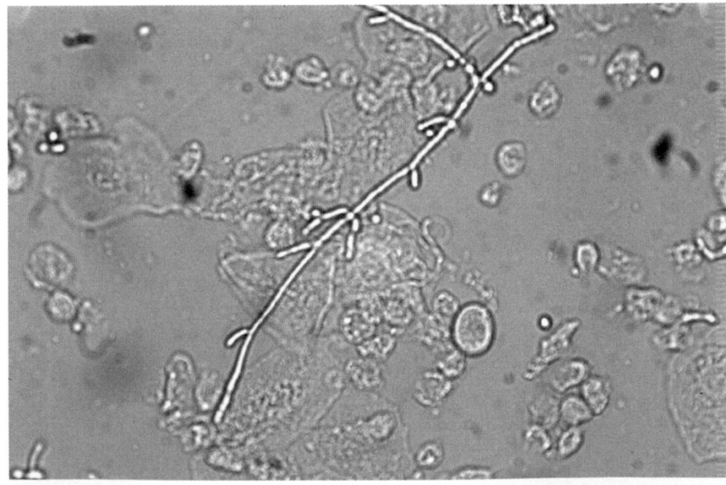

FIGURE 5.5. Wet-mount preparation showing budding pseudo-hyphal strand

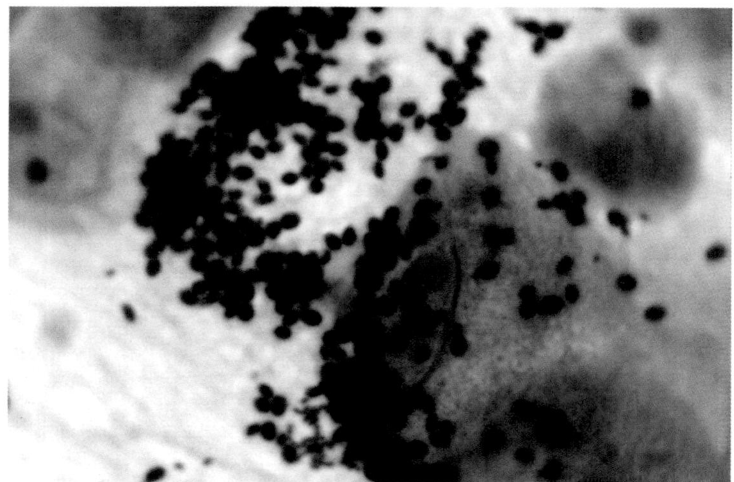

FIGURE 5.6. Gram stain of vaginal discharge due to *Candida glabrata* showing multiple spores without hyphae

Chapter 6
Other Causes of Vaginal Discharge

6.1 TRICHOMONIASIS

This has become less common in recent years and usually presents as quite a heavy yellow discharge associated with vulval and vaginal soreness. The motile trichomonads are easily seen on wet-mount microscopy (i.e. examination of a sample of vaginal discharge in a drop of normal saline under a cover slip; Figure 6.1); however, as this is rarely available in non-GU medicine settings, the diagnosis should be made by vaginal swab culture. This should be transported to the laboratory as soon as possible as the organism is quite friable.

Treatment is with oral metronidazole, preferably a 2 g stat dosage, although 400 mg b.d. for 5–7 days may be used. Metronidazole is better tolerated if taken with or after food, and alcohol should be avoided during treatment and for 24 hours afterward.

Most cases of trichomoniasis are sexually transmitted; sexual partners should therefore be assessed and treated. Men usually carry the infection without symptoms.

6.2 STREPTOCOCCAL INFECTION

Lancefield Group A and Group B streptococci are uncommon causes of vaginitis. Only approximately 50% of women with Group B infection report symptoms, usually vaginal soreness and irritation. Group A infection is less common but more likely to produce symptoms. There is frequently a marked vaginitis with a serosanguineous discharge.

6.3 DESQUAMATIVE VAGINITIS

This is an uncommon cause of discharge of unknown aetiology. The appearance is that of trichomoniasis, there being a marked vaginitis and profuse yellow discharge (Figure 6.2). Colposcopic examination of the vagina and cervix may show a macular pattern (as is often seen in trichomoniasis– so-called "strawberry cervix"). Gram stain and microscopy of the discharge shows an absence of lactobacilli with cocci-form bacteria and vaginal basal epithelial

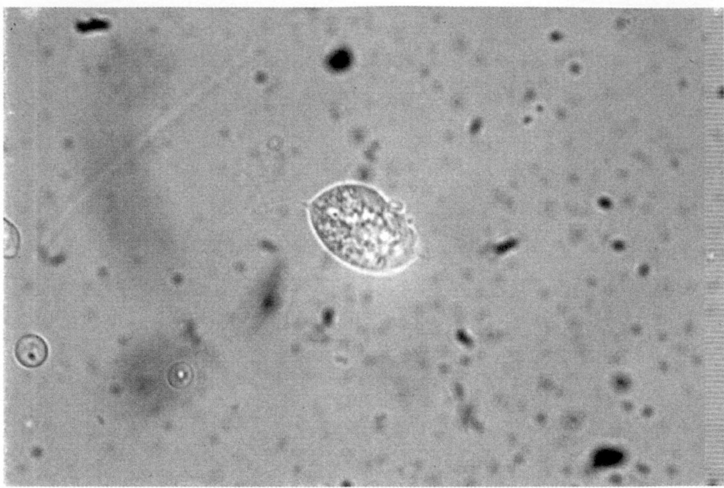

FIGURE 6.1. Wet-mount preparation showing a trichomonad (*Trichomonas vaginalis* infection)

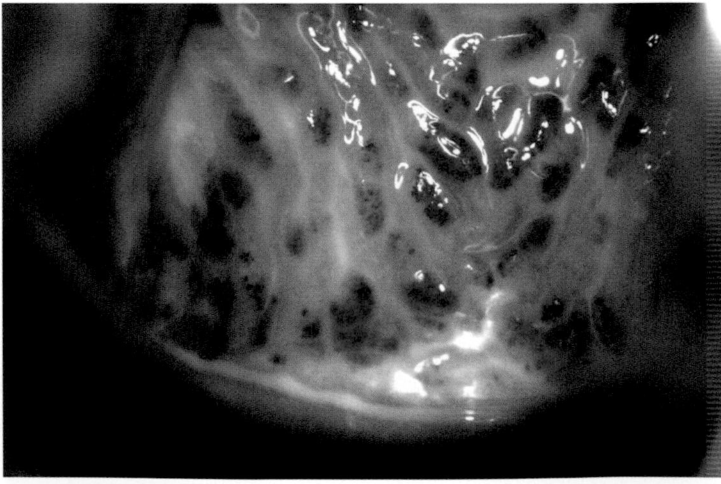

FIGURE 6.2. Macular vaginitis – seen in some cases of Trichomoniasis and desquamative vaginitis

cells present (as seen in a post menopausal woman with an atrophic vaginitis). There is often a good response to intravaginal Clindamycin cream.

6.4 FOREIGN OBJECTS

Liberal views on sexual experimentation have led to various devices becoming lodged or even lost in the vagina. Although the patient is usually only too aware that something has "gone missing," occasionally bits of "sex toys" can break off unknowingly and give rise to a vaginal discharge some days later.

More commonly a tampon can inadvertently be pushed deep into the vagina and be forgotten. After a few days this produces an unpleasant smelling discharge. Bits of tampons occasionally latch onto threads of an IUCD and later cause problems. These small pieces of cotton wool can often be very difficult to detect. Similarly, small fragments of toilet paper can be left at the entrance of the vagina following a hurried wipe after urination. Sexual activity can push these deep into the vagina only to produce a discharge after a few days.

Very occasionally condoms split during intercourse with the result that fragments of rubber may be retained in the vagina and eventually give rise to a malodorous discharge.

6.5 CERVICITIS

Cervical inflammation may cause a mucopurulent discharge which, although originating from the cervix, presents as a yellow vaginal discharge, sometimes blood stained.

6.5.1 Important Points

(1) Cervicitis is often difficult to distinguish from cervical ectopy as in both cases the cervix appears red to the naked eye. Indicators of cervicitis include mucopurulent secretions (Figure 6.3) and contact bleeding on touching the cervix with a cotton wool swab, for example when taking an endocervical swab for *Chlamydia* (not when scraping the cervix with a wooden spatula for cervical cytology). In GU medicine, cervical secretions are often examined under the microscope and the number of polymorphs present quantified. A count of greater than 30 polymorphs per high power field (HPF–×1000 magnification) is suggestive of a cervicitis.

A cervical ectopy may produce excessive mucus in the absence of infection. This can be treated by cryotherapy or

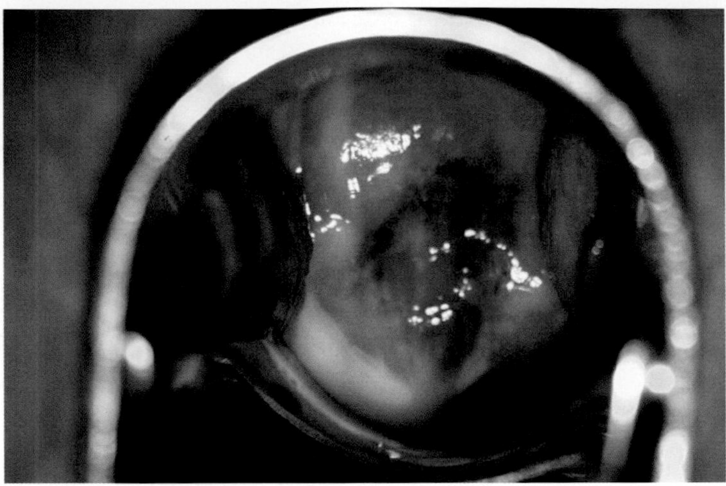

FIGURE 6.3. Mucopurulent cervicitis

diathermy but should only be considered when infection has been adequately checked for and discounted.

(2) *Chlamydia trachomatis* is the commonest cause of cervicitis in the UK. Remember to gently wipe the cervix clear of discharge before taking a swab for *Chlamydia*. Cellular material rather than mucus is required for diagnosis, although this is less of an issue with nucleic acid amplification tests than with enzyme immunoassays.

(3) Although gonorrhea is less common than *Chlamydia*, a swab should be taken from the cervix for *Neisseria gonorrhoeae* culture. The gonococcus is a fragile organism and therefore the sample must be transported to the laboratory as soon as possible; if there is likely to be an overnight delay then keep the swab at room temperature rather than in the refrigerator. Women with suspected gonorrhea should ideally be referred to GU medicine. The appropriate swabs from the cervix (not vagina), urethra, rectum, and pharynx (if appropriate) can then be taken and plated directly on to specific media and incubated prior to transport to the laboratory. Owing to the anatomical close proximity of anus and vagina, rectal infection may be present in the absence of a history of anal intercourse.

(4) In many cases no causative organism can be found and the diagnosis is one of "non-specific cervicitis" (the female

equivalent of "non-specific urethritis"). *Mycoplasma genitalium* may prove to be an important cause of cervicitis although currently this is a difficult organism to identify by routine microbiological testing.

6.5.2 Management of Cervicitis

Non-specific cervicitis and chlamydial infection should be treated with a tetracycline (e.g. doxycycline 100 mg bd for 7–10 days), erythromycin 500 mg b.d. (a 14-day course is usually required to adequately treat a chlamydial infection), azithromycin 1 g stat or azithromycin 500 mg stat followed by 250 mg daily for 4 days (more effective than 1g dosage for *M. genitalium* infection). Sexual partners should be assessed for urethritis; this is often asymptomatic. Failure to treat partners may lead to reinfection.

As mentioned above, patients with suspected gonorrhea should be referred to GU medicine for treatment, follow-up, and contact tracing (partner notification). If the diagnosis of gonorrhea has been confirmed by culture and there is a delay before the patient can be seen by GU medicine, consider treating with oral cefixime 400 mg stat and then refer to GU medicine for follow-up and contact tracing.

Penicillin- and ciprofloxacin-resistant gonorrhea is now seen in the UK, hence the recent move to using cephalosporins (oral cefixime and i.m. ceftriaxone are the favored choices). Intramuscular spectinomycin may be required for multiple resistant gonococcal infections but we are now moving into specialist territory. Most laboratories will provide details of antibiotic sensitivities for their gonococcal isolates.

Prescribing a 10-day course of tetracycline in addition to antigonococcal treatment to cover possible co-infection with *Chlamydia* is to be recommended.

6.6 PHYSIOLOGICAL DISCHARGE

Many women present with excessive vaginal discharge for which no infective cause can be found. In some cases this will be an increased awareness or a true increase in volume of normal vaginal secretions. Desquamated vaginal epithelial cells, cervical mucus, and transudated fluid from the vaginal mucosa are the main constituents of normal vaginal secretions and the amount produced may vary with the phase of the menstrual cycle. It is worth emphasizing that physiological discharge should be diagnosed only when both microscopy and culture of vaginal and cervical secretions prove negative; a clinical judgment is insufficient. Explaining the nature of the discharge and providing reassurance that no infection is present is often all that is required in the way of management. If the discharge is particularly troublesome, gentle douching with a povidone-iodine solution may be considered; because of the increased risk of pelvic infection associated with douching, it is important to ensure that infection is absent, in particular bacterial vaginosis and *Chlamydia*.

Some women with cervical ectopy produce an excessive amount of mucus and will often describe their discharge as "thick and stringy." Non-infected cervical mucus is clear or white; yellow mucus is highly suggestive of infection. Irrespective of the clinical findings the appropriate swabs must be taken to check for infection (see above) in addition to cervical cytology, if this has not been performed recently. Treatment with cryotherapy or diathermy should be considered once infection and cervical pathology have been excluded.

Chapter 7
A General Approach to the Management of Vaginal Discharge

It would be impractical, and indeed unnecessary, to refer all women with an abnormal vaginal discharge to GU medicine. Many women self-diagnose "thrush" and approach their GP requesting a repeat prescription of antifungals without investigation or examination. This is not an ideal approach to management. Confirmatory vaginal swabs should be taken on at least some occasions and if this is considered "difficult," for whatever reasons, then a GU medicine referral is advisable. There is also some concern that the availability of topical anti-"thrush" treatments without prescription may considerably delay some women from seeking professional help.

There are a few other points worth considering when deciding whether to refer a patient to GU medicine.

(1) In addition to obtaining optimal specimens for culture, microscopy of vaginal, cervical, and urethral secretions is performed routinely in all GU medicine clinics which enables the clinician to make, in many cases, an immediate diagnosis. Microscopy is an invaluable method of assessing the general health of the vagina and cervix. For example, a woman with symptomatic discharge showing a predominance of lactobacilli on the vaginal Gram stain, a normal cervical Gram stain and negative vaginal and cervical cultures, is most likely to have a physiological discharge.

(2) The two commonest causes of vaginal discharge seen in general practice and amongst attenders at GU medicine are candidiasis and bacterial vaginosis, neither of which are sexually transmitted. Microscopy of vaginal secretions is essential to accurately diagnose bacterial vaginosis; high vaginal swab culture is of no use.

(3) There are a few key questions that may give a clue to the diagnosis:
   - Irritation or soreness is suggestive of candidiasis.
   - A malodorous discharge is suggestive of bacterial vaginosis.
   - Intermenstrual bleeding or pelvic discomfort, a recent change of sexual partner, and the use of non-barrier contraception increase the likelihood of sexually transmitted infection.

(4) Which swabs to take. A Stuart's swab for microbiological culture is usually adequate to detect genital tract pathogens. It is important that the swab reaches the laboratory as soon as possible: *Trichomonas vaginalis* and the gonococcus are particularly delicate and may not survive an overnight delay before reaching specific culture media.

    Keep genital specimens for *T. vaginalis* culture at room temperature and swabs for *Neisseria gonorrhoeae* culture in the refrigerator if there is likely to be a delay before reaching the laboratory.

If gonorrhea is considered a possible diagnosis, the patient should be referred to GU medicine so that the appropriate swabs may be taken (i.e. urethral, cervical, rectal, and pharyngeal but NOT vaginal), plated on to the appropriate culture media and incubated prior to transport to the laboratory.

Chlamydia trachomatis is usually diagnosed by NAAT or antigen detection methods, such as the EIA. Wipe the cervix clear of vaginal secretions before taking an endocervical sample (i.e. a sample from the columnar epithelium) and remember that cellular material rather than mucus is required for diagnosis, although this is less of an issue for NAAT.

A 1–2 day delay in transport should not adversely affect the results. It is worth emphasizing that even with a perfectly taken clinical specimen the currently available EIA tests for *Chlamydia* may yield false positive or false negative results. Many laboratories will routinely retest positive samples using a different detection method from the original test. A positive result on both tests is likely to indicate a true infection. The significance of equivocal results must be judged on clinical merit. As our microbiology colleagues inform us, no test is 100% sensitive, sometimes a difficult concept to get over to our patients.

Bacterial vaginosis cannot be diagnosed from a vaginal swab unless a Gram stain is prepared.

Guidelines for the management of vaginal discharge are summarized in Table 7.1.

TABLE 7.1. Diagnosis and management of vaginal discharge

	Possible Diagnosis
1. Take a history	
Any suggestion of sexually transmitted infection (e.g. recent change of sexual partner)	
Vulval irritation or soreness	Candidiasis or trichomoniasis
Malodor	Bacterial vaginosis
2. Examination	
Vulval/vaginal erythema	Candidiasis or trichomoniasis
"Lumpy" or "curd-like" discharge	Candidiasis
Smooth, homogeneous, slightly frothy discharge	Bacterial vaginosis
Moderately heavy yellow discharge	Trichomoniasis; cervicitis
Yellow cervical mucus ± contact bleeding on gently swabbing the cervix	Cervicitis
3. Investigations	
(a) Vaginal swab (e.g. Stuart's) (probably not worth taking if >24 h delay before arriving in laboratory) (Keep swabs for *T. vaginalis* culture at room temperature and swabs for *N. gonorrhoeae* culture in the refrigerator)	Candidiasis, trichomoniasis, streptococcal infection
(b) Second vaginal swab	
Roll gently onto microscope slide	
AIR dry	
Ask laboratory to Gram stain	Bacterial vaginosis
Before discarding, drop 1–5% KOH onto swab and sniff	
→ pronounced "fish-like" odor – positive "amine" test	Bacterial vaginosis
If sexually transmitted infection a possibility or clinical suspicion of cervicitis → refer to GU medicine clinic	
If patient unwilling or impractical to attend:	
(a) Cervical swab: Stuart's (send to laboratory as soon as possible)	Gonorrhea
(b) Second cervical swab (special test kits available which contain appropriate swab and transport medium)	*Chlamydia*
Also consider taking urethral swabs for	

(Continued)

TABLE 7.1. (Continued)

Chlamydia and gonorrhea in conjunction with cervical specimens (see text)

4. Management summary

Diagnosis	*Treatment*
Candidiasis	A topical imidazole (pessaries and cream), oral fluconazole 150 mg stat, oral itraconazole 200 mg bd for 1 day
Bacterial vaginosis	Oral metronidazole, e.g. 2 g suspension stat; 200 mg tds for 7 days; 400 mg bd for 5 days Intravaginal 0.75% metronidazole gel daily for 5 days Intravaginal 2% clindamycin cream for 7 days Oral clindamycin 300 mg bd for 7 days
Trichomoniasis	Oral metronidazole, e.g. 2 g suspension stat or 400 mg bd for 5–7 days Sexual partners should be assessed and treated
Chlamydia	Tetracyclines (e.g. doxycycline 100 mg bd for 7–10 days) Erythromycin (500 mg bd for 14 days) Azithromycin 1 g stat Strongly consider referral to GU medicine for follow-up and contact tracing
Gonorrhoea	Cefixime 400 mg oral stat Ceftriaxone 250 mg intra-muscular stat Patients found to have gonorrhoea should ideally be referred to GU medicine for follow-up and contact tracing

(bd, twice daily; tds, three times daily; GU, genitourinary; stat, once only.)

Chapter 8
Vulval Problems

Vulval disease is common and although most of the conditions presenting in general practice are straightforward, a significant number of women pose rather more of a diagnostic and management problem.

The following are the important points to consider:

(1) What are the predominant symptoms: irritation, soreness or burning?
Is there an urge to scratch or is the skin too sore?
Is the whole vulva affected or are symptoms localized to one particular area?
(2) Is there a personal or family history of allergy?
(3) Any history of skin problems, for example dermatitis/eczema, psoriasis, lichen planus?
(4) Which soap is used for cleansing the genital area? Are bubble-bath, hygiene sprays, etc. used?
(5) Are symptoms related to the time in the menstrual cycle or brought on by coitus?

Although candidiasis is the commonest cause of vulval irritation, this diagnosis should be reconsidered if vaginal swabs fail to grow the fungus and there is no response to antifungal treatment. If there is doubt, consider using a longer course of an oral antifungal (e.g. itraconazole or fluconazole) as a diagnostic test. If there is no clinical response to antifungals in spite of *Candida* being isolated on culture, ask the laboratory to identify the *Candida* spp., as some of the more unusual strains (e.g. *Candida glabrata*) may be resistant to the commonly used imidazole and triazole preparations.

Although the vulva may be affected by a variety of skin conditions, the clinical features are often modified by secondary infection, scratching (causing lichenification or skin thickening), or by previous treatments. Examination of the scalp, nails, elbows, and mouth may provide useful clues to the diagnosis.

8.1 VULVAL IRRITATION

Conditions that may present with vulval irritation include the following:

(1) Candidiasis (see above, Chapter 5 and Figures 5.1 to 5.3).

(2) Human papillomavirus (HPV) infection (see also Chapter 18). Genital warts can cause slight irritation and when they first appear may be quite difficult to identify without some form of magnification, such as a colposcope. (Note: Anal warts may present as pruritis ani; beware the diagnosis of hemorrhoids without careful examination!) Vulval intraepithelial neoplasia (VIN, Figure 8.1) is strongly associated with HPV type 16 infection and often presents as white or off-white, flat or papular lesions, most commonly affecting the labia minora and perineum. Lesions are multifocal in 70% of women and cause irritation in just under two-thirds. Biopsy should be considered to confirm the diagnosis and stage the lesion (VIN I, VIN II, or VIN III). VIN has the potential to progress to squamous cell carcinoma, particularly in the more mature woman, and therefore careful follow-up is advisable. In addition, as VIN is associated with dysplasia elsewhere in the genital tract, it is important to ensure that cervical

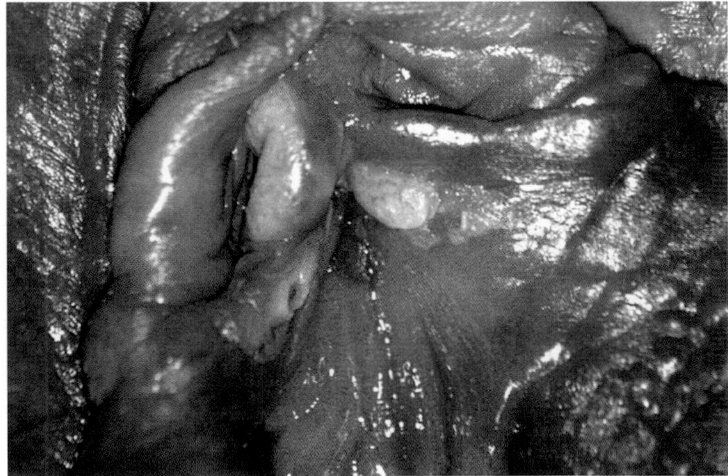

FIGURE 8.1. Vulval intraepithelial neoplasia (VIN)

cytology, and if possible colposcopy, is performed on a regular basis, ideally annually.

(3) Genital herpes (see also Chapter 17). Some women report vulval irritation before ulcers appear. With primary genital herpes, the irritation is soon superseded by increasing soreness and subsequently ulceration and vulval edema. The typical blisters are fragile and often missed. A history of a "flu-like" illness or sore throat prior to the onset of the vulval symptoms is often a helpful diagnostic clue. Women presenting with primary genital herpes often give a history of supposed "thrush" that has worsened whilst using antifungals.

In recurrent herpes, the vulval lesions may be tiny and easily overlooked unless the patient or examining clinician is alert to the possible diagnosis. Examination with a magnifying glass or colposcope can be helpful in these cases.

(4) Trichomoniasis. *Trichomonas vaginalis* usually causes a vulvovaginitis associated with an increased vaginal discharge. Diagnosis is by wet-mount microscopy or culture (see Chapter 6, Figure 6.1).

(5) Streptococcal infection. Although both Lancefield Group A and Group B streptococci may cause a vulvovaginitis, this is uncommon and vulval infection usually occurs secondarily to an already damaged vulval skin, for example from dermatitis. Vulval erysipelas is usually associated with Group A streptococci and presents as pronounced labial swelling and erythema which may progress to necrosis.

(6) Dermatoses. These are not uncommon and often involve the labia majora and perineum.
   (a) Seborrheic dermatitis (Figure 8.2). Look for evidence elsewhere, such as on the face, chest, and scalp.
   (b) Contact dermatitis. There is often a history of allergies or family history of atopy. Check whether any creams or lotions are being applied to the genital area. Latex allergy usually presents as vaginal soreness after using condoms. Seminal fluid, KY jelly, or spermicide allergy presents as postcoital vaginal discomfort sometimes associated with vulval edema. Scented soaps, bubble-baths, hygiene sprays, antimicrobial creams, and anesthetic hemorrhoid creams are potential sensitizers.
   (c) Lichen simplex (Figure 8.3). Some degree of skin thickening or lichenification is common after chronic scratching. Treatment with a moderately potent topical steroid is often required.

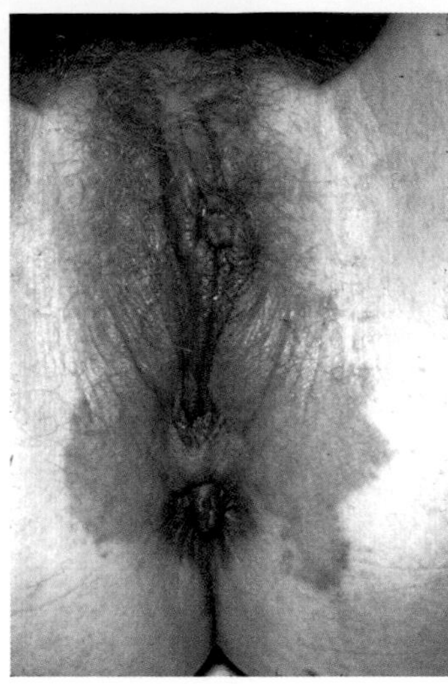

FIGURE 8.2. Seborrhoeic dermatitis

(d) Lichen planus (Figure 8.4). Look for evidence elsewhere, particularly in the mouth. Erosive lichen planus is a variant that may present with severe vulvitis and vaginitis.

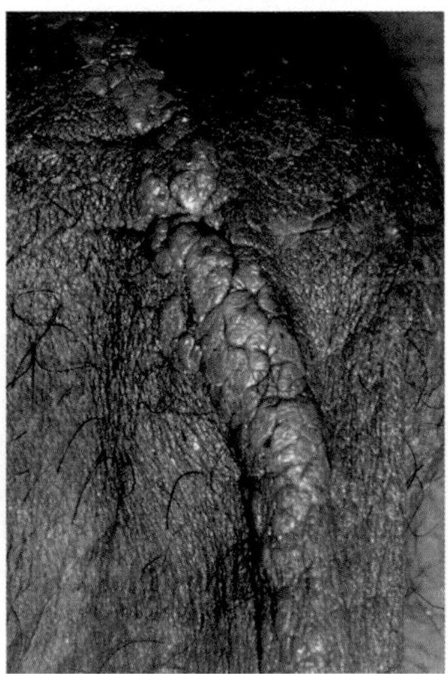

FIGURE 8.3. Lichen simplex

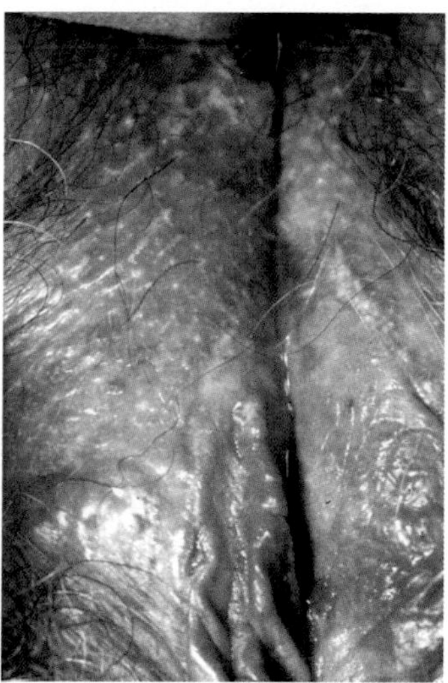

FIGURE 8.4. Lichen planus

(e) Psoriasis (Figure 8.5). Look for evidence elsewhere, including nail pitting, and ask about family history. Lesions in the genital area may not appear typical as the scale is often lost leaving a red, glazed epithelium.

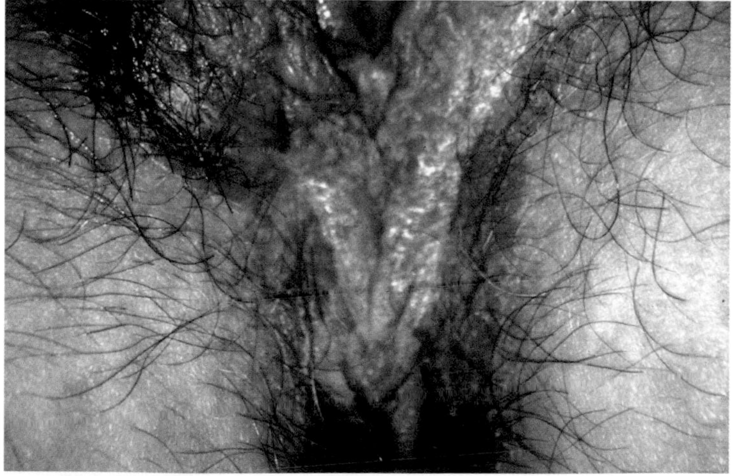

FIGURE 8.5. Psoriasis

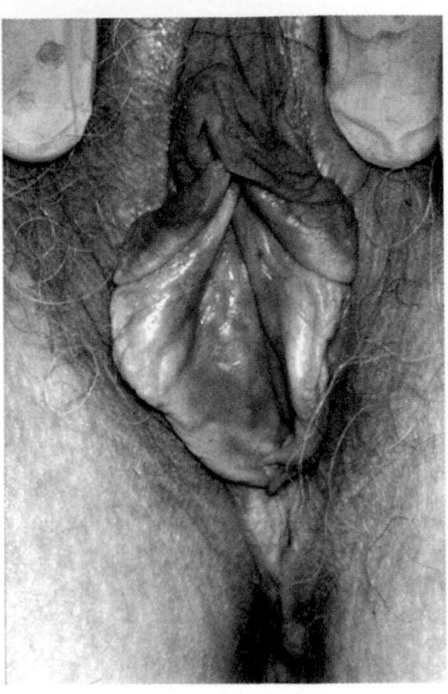

FIGURE 8.6. Lichen sclerosus – atrophic changes

(f) Lichen sclerosus (Figure 8.6). Commonly affects the perianal and genital regions in children and adults. Often presents with irritation and less commonly soreness. Sexual intercourse can be painful either because of friction damaging the fragile vulval skin or secondary to tightening of the vaginal introitus resulting from post-inflammatory scarring. In the early stages the skin appears white and slightly thinned sometimes with small, superficial erosions and "blood blisters." Untreated, the inflammatory process may lead to resorption of the labia minora and clitoris and narrowing of the introitus (Figure 8.7). Active disease should be treated initially with a potent topical steroid (e.g. clobetasol propionate). Long-term follow-up is recommended because of the small risk (up to 4%) of developing squamous cell carcinoma.

8.1.1 A Short note about Topical Steroids

Patients are often concerned that topical steroids will damage the skin, particularly in the genital region, and may therefore fail to treat themselves adequately. It is worth reassuring patients that steroid creams and ointments are safe to use under clinical supervision and are required, sometimes in high strength and for long periods of time, to adequately treat skin problems. Not too much cream need be applied and suggesting to the patient that a tube

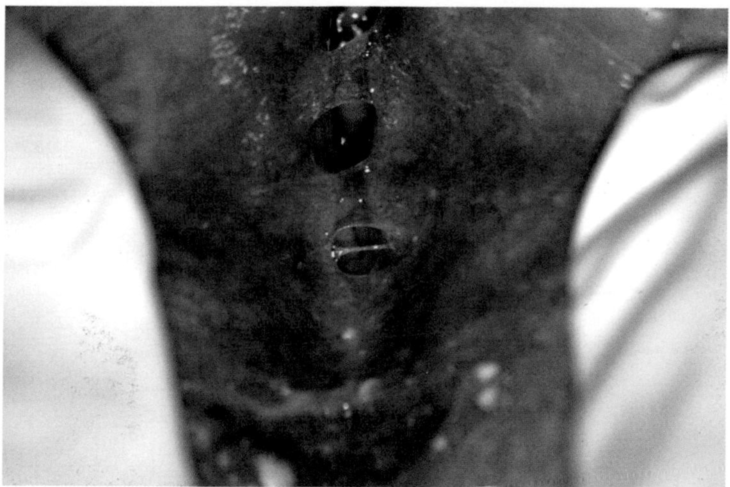

FIGURE 8.7. Lichen sclerosus – showing adhesion formation between the labia

should last a year or two may help to avoid over treatment. Creams sometimes sting a little more on application than ointments but may be easier to apply to mucosal surfaces. Combined steroid and anti-infective preparations may be required to treat genital dermatoses but be alert to hypersensitivity reactions to the topical antibiotic components (e.g. neomycin, tetracycline). Some conditions (e.g. lichen sclerosus) should be initially treated with a potent topical steroid and then a weaker preparation substituted after a few weeks when symptoms have improved.

8.2 VULVAL SORENESS OR TENDERNESS

All of the above conditions may cause soreness in addition to or rather than irritation.

8.2.1 Vulvar Vestibulitis

This is an important, frequently misdiagnosed, or missed condition that causes pain on sexual intercourse, particularly penetration. Tampons may also be too uncomfortable to use. It would be reasonable to say that all women presenting with insertional dyspareunia should be considered to have vulvar vestibulitis until proven otherwise. The condition presents as small areas of localized erythema (Figure 8. 8) and tenderness at the introitus, classically over the vestibular gland openings at

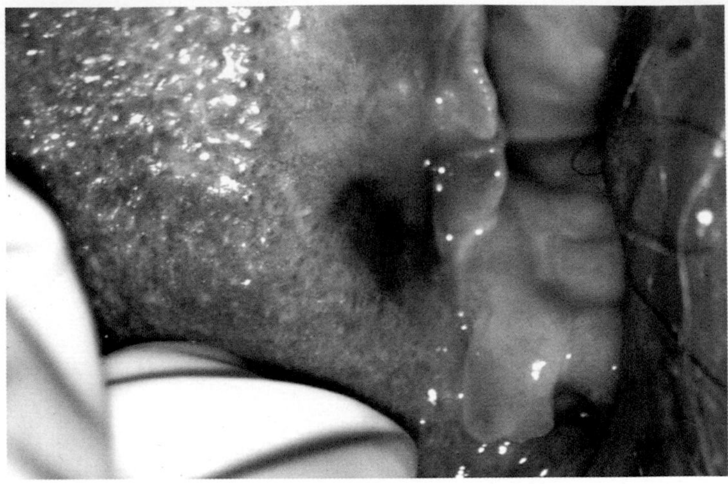

FIGURE 8.8. Vulvar vestibulitis – area of erythema at introital 7 o'clock position

the 5 o'clock and 7 o'clock positions. Some form of magnification, such as a colposcope, will often be required to see the lesions adequately. The cause of vulvar vestibulitis is currently unknown. Some women experience pain from coitarche whilst others give a history of years of pain-free sexual intercourse. A variety of treatments have been used in this condition with, unfortunately, often poor response. These include topical steroids, topical estrogens, intralesional triamcinolone, cryotherapy, and laser ablation. Modified vestibulectomy has produced good results in some studies but patients need to be selected with care. Some women show marked introital sensitivity, with light touch with a cotton wool swab invoking marked tenderness (allodynia). Low dose amitriptyline (10 mg initially slowly increasing to 50 mg or 75 mg, if tolerated) or pregabilin can prove helpful in these cases.

8.2.2 Posterior Fourchette Tear

Posterior fourchette tears cause pain during sexual intercourse, sometimes associated with bleeding. Examination with a colposcope may be required to make the diagnosis as the tears are often very small. Although a mild strength combined steroid/ antibacterial cream may prove helpful, some women are prone to recurrences. Tearing is sometimes associated with

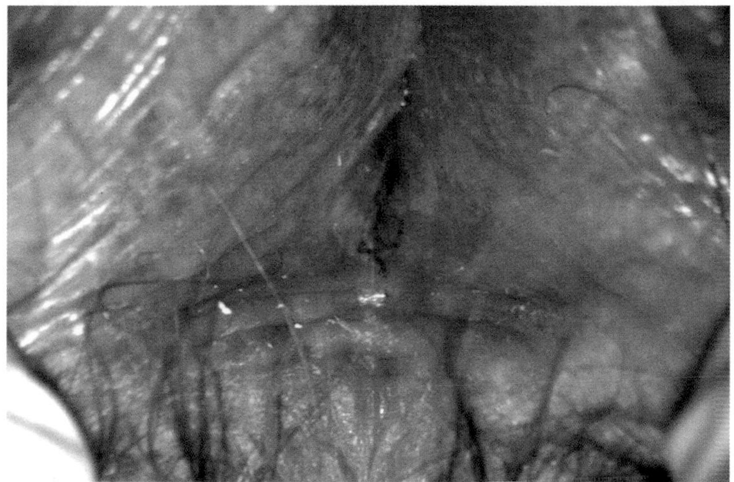

FIGURE 8.9. Posterior fourchette tear

a bridge of skin at this site, in which case surgical removal (e.g. modified Fenton's procedure) should be considered (Figure 8.9).

8.3 VULVAL BURNING

"Essential vulvodynia" or "dysesthetic vulvodynia" is the term used to describe symptoms of vulval burning with a normal appearing epithelium. Pudendal neuralgia is an important cause with some patients demonstrating diminished sensation in the sacral sensory distribution. Benign sacral meningeal cysts have been reported to cause genital pain and burning in both men and women; the diagnosis being made by magnetic resonance imaging of the lumbosacral spine. I would however suggest a neurological referral or alternative specialist opinion before requesting MRI scans on your patients with genital pain.

In the majority of patients, however, no obvious physical cause can be found for their symptoms in which case psychological issues should be considered and addressed.

Management may include the use of 'pain modifiers', such as low to medium dose amitriptyline, prothiaden or fluoxetine, pregabalin, gabapentin, hypnosis, acupuncture, transcutaneous electrical nerve simulation (TENS) or caudal injection. Amitriptyline or pregabalin are useful first line options.

8.4 OTHER VULVAL CONDITIONS

8.4.1 Vulval Edema

The lax vulval skin is prone to edema and is particularly associated with infections such as herpes, candidiasis, and syphilis, although the latter is uncommon in women in the UK nowadays. Edema is an occasional feature of contact dermatitis and has been reported following intercourse in women with semen allergy. Vulval edema may be a presenting sign of Crohn's disease and intrapelvic pathology.

8.4.2 Angiokeratomata

These small lesions usually appear on the labia majora as tiny, often multiple, bright red vascular spots (Figure 8.10). They may increase in number and size with age and are harmless.

8.4.3 Melanocytic Naevi

These may appear anywhere on the vulva or perineum and have the same characteristics as naevi elsewhere on the body.

See also Chapters 17 and 18.

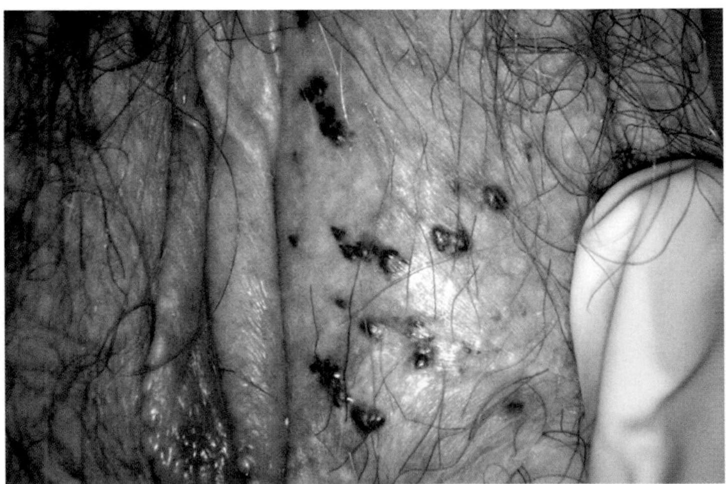

FIGURE 8.10. Angiokeratomata

8.5 IMPORTANT MANAGEMENT POINTS FOR VULVAL DISEASE

- Vulval moistness may increase the risk of secondary infection with yeasts or bacteria. Advise patients to dry the skin thoroughly after washing, if possible with a hair dryer on cool setting. Avoid tight clothing and try to ventilate the area as much as sociably possible.
- Even with careful attention, secondary infection of genital dermatoses may occur. Treatment with a combined anti-infective and steroidal preparation should be considered.
- Although creams are often easier to apply to the genital epithelium, they may sting a little more than ointments.
- Soap, bubble-bath, shower gel, and feminine washes should be avoided. Many women find aqueous cream or emulsifying ointment useful as soap substitutes for cleansing. Applying cold cream from the refrigerator can be particularly soothing.
- Vulval biopsy may be required to accurately diagnose skin dermatoses. The application of lignocaine/prilocaine cream prior to injecting local anesthetic makes this a painless and generally well-tolerated procedure.
- All painful vulval conditions have the potential to cause a secondary vaginismus that can often persist after the original complaint has settled. This will require appropriate treatment and follow-up. (see also Chapter 22)
- Vulval disease is often chronic and inevitably affects relationships and leads to a degree of psychological morbidity. Psychological support is therefore an important part of the management of these patients and should be considered along with treatment aimed at the physical component of the condition.
- The diagnosis and management of vulval disease can be difficult and may, in some cases, require the assistance of a clinician with a specific interest in the vulva. Many hospitals now run "vulva clinics" where specialists in GU medicine, dermatology and gynecology offer a combined opinion. This is the ideal approach to managing vulval disease.

Chapter 9
Frequency–Dysuria Syndrome

Frequency and dysuria in the female are usually due to the following:

- Cystitis
- Urethritis/urethral syndrome
- Vulvitis.

Women with vulvitis will often complain of more generalized vulval irritation or soreness in addition to dysuria. The urinary symptoms are due to urine touching an inflamed labial epithelium or due to peri-urethral inflammation.

It is impossible to distinguish between cystitis and urethritis/urethral syndrome by symptoms alone. As a useful rule of thumb, if urine dipstix testing is entirely normal and the midstream urine culture is negative or shows sterile pyuria, consider urethritis/ urethral syndrome.

9.1 CYSTITIS

In cystitis, the MSU should contain $>10^5$ uropathogens per ml. This criterion was originally established for diagnosing acute pyelonephritis and several studies have since suggested that a lower bacterial count of between 10^3 and 10^5 per ml indicates bladder infection, particularly when Gram-positive bacteria (e.g. *Staphylococcus saprophyticus*) or atypical organisms (e.g. *Proteus*) are involved. Studies have reported that between one-third to one-half of women with bacterial cystitis have "low-count" bacteruria. The commonest causes of cystitis are *E. coli*, *S. saprophyticus*, *Proteus mirabilis*, *Klebsiella pneumoniae*, and *Enterobacter* spp.

9.2 URETHRITIS/URETHRAL SYNDROME

Women with frequency and dysuria and urine containing $<10^3$ uropathogens per ml with or without pyuria are usually diagnosed as having "urethral syndrome." Some will have a true urethritis that may be diagnosed by finding polymorphs on a Gram-stained urethral smear, an investigation often performed in GU medicine.

Chlamydia trachomatis is the most important organism to consider. Appropriate swabs should be taken from the cervix in addition to the urethra as infection at both sites is common.

Although some studies have suggested that fastidious bacteria colonizing the vulval vestibule, such as lactobacilli and diphtheroids, may occasionally infect the urethra and produce frequency and dysuria, this continues to be a topic of debate.

Other causes of urethral syndrome include the following:

- Gonorrhea (very unusual to present with frequency and/or dysuria as the only symptoms)
- Herpes (usually associated with vulval or periurethral ulceration)
- Trichomoniasis (usually associated with an increased vaginal discharge)
- HPV infection (a small intrameatal/distal urethral genital wart).

9.3 INVESTIGATION OF FREQUENCY – DYSURIA

Dipstix testing and looking at the urine are useful first-line tests. Cystitis is highly unlikely if the urine looks clear and dipstix testing is negative for nitrites, leucocytes, blood, and protein.

As a general rule, consider sending an MSU for microscopy and culture if dipstix testing is positive for nitrites, leucocytes, blood, and protein, although bear in mind that contamination with vaginal discharge may yield positive dipstix results for leucocytes, protein, or blood. Women with recurrent symptoms should ideally have tests repeated at the onset of each symptomatic episode.

If these tests prove negative, consider the following:

- Checking for chlamydial infection by taking urethral *and* cervical swabs (if either are positive, sexual partners *must* be assessed)
- Taking a vaginal swab for *Trichomonas vaginalis* and *Candida* culture
- Referring to GU medicine for colposcopic examination of the urethral meatus, distal urethra, and periurethral area for evidence of tiny genital warts, small herpetic ulcers, or a localized area of vulvitis. Examination should be performed when symptoms are present.

9.3.1 Recurrent Frequency – Dysuria

- Women with recurrent episodes of proven cystitis should be referred to urology for investigation of urinary tract pathology.
- Some women with a "low-set," almost intravaginal, urethral meatus are prone to recurrent postcoital cystitis. Attacks may be prevented by urinating directly after intercourse or by using prophylactic single dose antibiotics pre- or post-coitus.
- Advise wiping from "front-to-back" after defecation.
- Consider a 10–14 day course of a tetracycline. The currently available EIA tests for diagnosing chlamydial infection are not 100% sensitive and so a false negative result should be considered. Nucleic acid amplification tests are more sensitive and hence reliable but a course of tetracycline is still worth trying, remembering that doxycycline has an anti-inflammatory as well as antibacterial action.
- Cranberry juice may have a protective effect against recurrent urinary tract infection in women at risk of developing such infections. Cranberry juice has been shown to interfere with bacterial adherence in vitro and also may act by eliminating uropathogenic bacteria from the gut.
- Urethral dilatation or urethrotomy will benefit some women.
- The use of intravaginal estrogen may help to prevent recurrent urinary tract infections in postmenopausal women.

A number of women suffer chronic urinary symptoms for which no obvious cause can be found. Underlying psychological issues should be carefully sought and discussed openly with the patient. Suggesting that symptoms are "in the mind" is usually unhelpful whereas an approach that recognizes the symptoms as real and attempts to help the patient to "de-focus" the mind from the urinary tract by way of hypnosis, behaviour therapy, meditation or low-moderate dose antidepressants, as used for chronic pain relief, may prove helpful.

Chapter 10
Pelvic Pain

Women with acute, severe pelvic pain are most appropriately assessed by a gynecologist. Chronic or recurrent pelvic pain can be notoriously difficult to diagnose and manage and although many women will eventually require a gynecological assessment, GU medicine can play an important role in assessing patients for evidence of genital infection. Referral to GU medicine may therefore be an appropriate first step for women with pelvic discomfort or pain and if no evidence of infection is found gynecological referral should then be considered.

Pelvic inflammatory disease is difficult to diagnose without the aid of laparoscopy and many women are unfortunately labeled as having PID on insufficient clinical grounds. This can lead to a great deal of anxiety, particularly regarding infertility. It is impractical to offer laparoscopy to all women with pelvic pain and if PID is considered a possible diagnosis then the uncertainty of the diagnosis should be discussed with the patient, the appropriate genital swabs taken, appropriate antibiotics prescribed, male sexual partners assessed for asymptomatic urethritis and chlamydial infection, and the patient reassessed after treatment.

Chlamydia trachomatis is the commonest cause of PID in the UK and although many women will present with increased vaginal discharge and pelvic discomfort/pain, there is now good evidence to suggest that *Chlamydia* can produce subclinical pelvic infection. As with classical PID, subclinical infection may cause tubal damage and subsequent infertility.

Gonorrhoea is less common in the U.K. than chlamydial infection but the diagnosis must be considered in all women with presumed pelvic infection. *Mycoplasma genitalium* has also been recently recognised as a sexually transmitted pathogen, capable of causing urethritis, cervicitis and pelvic inflammatory disease.

10.1 DIAGNOSIS AND MANAGEMENT OF PELVIC INFLAMMATORY DISEASE

(1) The following swabs should be taken:

(a) Vaginal and cervical swabs for Gram staining and microscopy. Unfortunately these are rarely performed in settings other than GU medicine clinics in the UK. Most PID results from an ascending lower genital tract infection, so there is often evidence of an abnormal vaginal microflora, such as bacterial vaginosis, or of a cervicitis. Mucopurulent cervical secretions provide clinical evidence of cervicitis; however, this is not always easy to assess unless there is excellent lighting and an experienced eye (see also chapter 6 page 29). Confirmation can be made by examining a Gram-stained smear of cervical secretions by microscopy: the presence of >30–40 polymorphs per high power field (HPF – x1000 magnification) is highly suggestive of cervicitis. A normal lactobacilli-predominant vaginal flora and the absence of cervicitis make PID a less likely diagnosis.

(b) Cervical swabs (NOT vaginal) for *Chlamydia* detection and *Neisseria gonorrhoeae* culture. Remember that organisms may be present in the uterus and fallopian tubes in spite of negative cervical cultures. Tests are currently not routinely available for diagnosing *Mycoplasma genitalium* infection.

(2) A raised ESR and peripheral white blood cell count are often present in acute PID but are non-specific and therefore provide little clinical guidance.

(3) Remember that the most important differential diagnoses for acute PID are acute appendicitis and ectopic pregnancy. Other conditions which may mimic PID include endometriosis, corpus luteum bleeding, urinary tract infection, mesenteric lymphadenitis, and ovarian tumor. The more common differential diagnoses of chronic pelvic pain include endometriosis, irritable bowel syndrome, and pelvic congestion.

(4) Treatment of PID should include antibiotics active against *Chlamydia*, anaerobes, and the gonococcus.

Possible oral combinations include the following:

- Doxycycline 100 mg bd + co-amoxiclav 500 mg tds

  or
- Ofloxacin 400 mg bd + metronidazole 400 mg bd + ciprofloxacin 500 mg bd

  or
- Doxycycline 100 mg bd + metronidazole 400 mg bd + cefixime 200 mg od.

At least 2–3 weeks of anti-chlamydial and anti-anaerobic treatment are recommended. Ciprofloxacin or cefixime may be stopped after 1 week. There is currently no evidence to suggest that treatment with non-steroidal anti-inflammatory drugs reduces the risk of tubal scarring.

(5) Advise bed rest and analgesia as required.

(6) It is imperative that sexual partners are assessed for evidence of urethritis and treated, otherwise recurrence is likely. Further attacks of PID increase the chances of infertility: following three episodes of PID there is a more than 50% chance of infertility. Urethritis is frequently asymptomatic in male contacts of women with PID, a point worth stressing to the patient.

(7) A number of women suffer chronic pelvic pain for which no obvious cause can be found. Underlying psychological issues should be carefully sought and discussed openly with the patient. Suggesting that symptoms are "in the mind" is usually unhelpful, whereas an approach that recognizes the symptoms as real and attempts to help the patient "de-focus" by way of hypnosis, meditation or low-dose antidepressants, as used for chronic pain relief, may prove helpful.

Chapter 11
Cytology and Colposcopy

Cervical cancer is in most cases a preventable disease and cervical cytology is an effective method of screening for abnormalities that have the potential to progress to cancer. The current UK National Guidelines for cervical screening are as follows:

- First smear at 25 years of age
- Three yearly smears between ages 25 and 49
- Five yearly smears between ages 50 and 64
- Smears recommended above the age of 65 if a recent abnormal smear or no screening performed since the age of 50.

Sexual health issues can be usefully discussed at the time of first cytology and screening for sexually acquired infections, in particular chlamydia, considered. For this reason, some clinicians are concerned at delaying screening until 25 years of age. From a cancer prevention perspective, the delay in initiating screening is certainly cost-effective as cervical cancer below the age of 25 is rare in the UK. In 2002, five deaths from cervical cancer were registered amongst women aged between 16 and 24 years of age.

Repeating cytology every 2 years is 50% more expensive than screening every 3 years. A study from the United States has shown that in a well screened population, three yearly screening would prevent virtually all cervical cancers prevented by annual screening with an additional 70000 smears and 400 colposcopic examinations being needed to prevent one extra cancer.

Extending the screening period after the age of 50 is based on data showing that the prevalence of CIN III and cervical cancer is very low beyond this age in a well-screened population.

Cervical cytology has an approximately 70% sensitivity for detecting cervical pathology and hence there is a need for an improvement in cervical screening technology. Liquid based cytology (LBC) has now replaced conventional cytology in the USA, UK and some other European countries. A Cervex brush (or similar sampling tool) is used to obtain the cervical sample and, instead of smearing on to a microscope slide, the brush is vigorously 'stirred' into a buffer solution to produce a suspension of cells. This is then used to produce a monolayer of cells, without the usual blood cells and other debris. These cleaner samples can be read more quickly and should increase the sensitivity for detecting pathological changes and reduce the number of inadequate samples. However, recent commentators have questioned the claims that LBC performs better than conventional cytology and have emphasised the need for large randomized controlled trails.

The use of HPV testing to improve on sensitivity and as a cost-effective means of triaging women for colposcopy is currently being studied. A positive result for one of the "high risk" HPV types (e.g. HPV 16 or 18) is known to generate patient anxiety and yet this often represents only a transient infection of no long-term consequence. Persistent infection or infection associated with dyskaryosis is of greater significance and it is likely that HPV testing will be used in conjunction with cytology as a means of identifying more accurately those women at risk of developing high grade dysplasia and cervical carcinoma. Women with persistent borderline or mildly abnormal smears and a positive result for high risk HPV types may be colposcoped earlier than if high risk HPV testing proved negative.

11.1 TAKING A SMEAR

Most of us will have passed through undergraduate training without proper instruction on how to take a cervical smear and occasionally the basic principles are forgotten, even by the most experienced clinician. There are three important points to consider:

(1) To obtain a "good" smear the cervix must be well visualized. This is an obvious point but not always followed. The following guidelines may help to make the procedure a little easier for both patient and practitioner.
  (a) Try to relax the patient.
  (b) Warm the speculum.
  (c) Use an appropriately sized speculum. A nulliparous woman in her early twenties usually requires a smaller speculum than a 40-year-old woman with five children. A very long speculum is occasionally required; it is well worthwhile keeping one or two in the surgery.
  (d) Insert the speculum gently and open slowly looking for the cervix as you proceed. Inserting the speculum completely before opening sometimes leads to the cervix

being passed and provides only a view of the anterior or posterior fornix. "Gently" is the key; a heavy hand leads to discomfort and may deter the patient from attending for gynecological examinations in the future.

(e) Good lighting is essential.

(2) Cervical dysplasia and neoplasia usually originate in the "transformation zone" adjacent to the "squamo-columnar junction" (see Figure 11.1). To help adequately sample this area a range of shapes of cervical spatulae and brushes are available (Figure 11.2). Pick the most appropriate device for the individual cervix. As a basic guide, if there is no obvious ectropion or ectopy, the squamo-columnar junction will be just at or inside the cervical os, then an Aylesbury spatula or "Cervex" sampler should provide an adequate sample. A cervical brush can also be used but ideally this should be in conjunction with a sample obtained by spatula. A "brush only" sample often contains too few squamous cells for adequate assessment. Brush and spatula samples may be spread on to different halves of the same slide. Take the brush sample last as the cells tend to dry out quickly, roll the brush over the slide and fix immediately. Combined 'brush and spatula' samples are usually required after cervical surgery (e.g. LLETZ (large loop excision of the transformation zone), laser, cone biopsy).

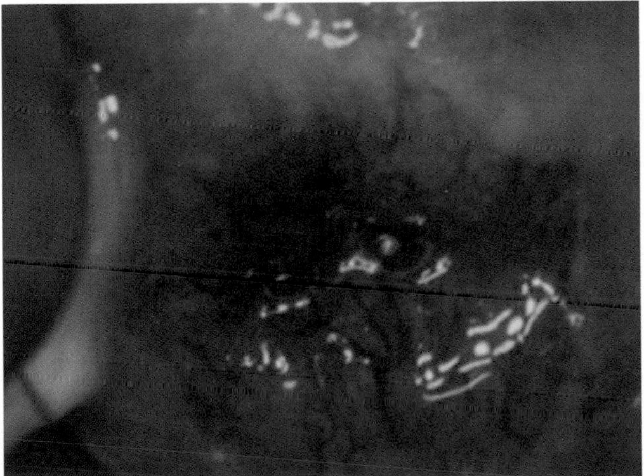

FIGURE 11.1. Cervical ectopy demonstrating well the squamo-columnar junction

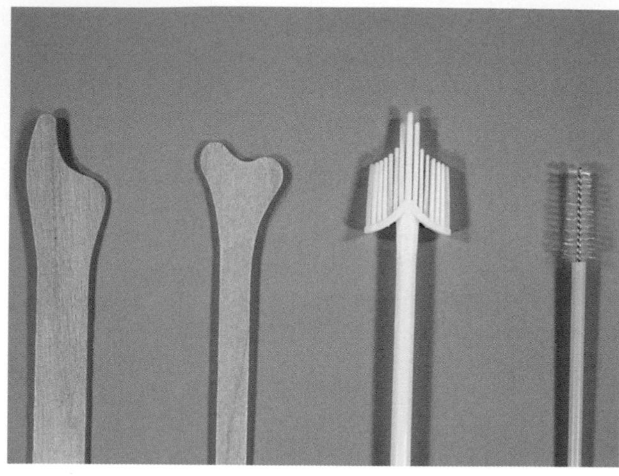

FIGURE 11.2. Cervical spatulae and brushes for cervical cytology (a) Aylesbury spatula (b) Ayre's spatula (c) Cervex® brush (d) Cytobrush®

An Aylesbury spatula should also be suitable if there is a small ectropion whereas an Ayre's spatula is probably best reserved for the cervix with a moderately sized or large ectropion. The entire squamo-columnar junction must be sampled which in some women requires quite firm pressure if the posterior aspect of the junction is to be reached. Two or three 360° turns usually picks up sufficient material combined with a lateral sweep if the ectropion is particularly large. Spread the material evenly over the microscope slide and fix immediately. If there is only a scanty amount of material on the slide, resample with a "Cervex" brush or one of the newer plastic/foam bendable devices, again remembering to aim for the squamo-columnar junction.

Mention on the cytology form if you have used a cervical brush because it often picks up glandular components that can give the cytologist the false impression of cervical pathology.

It is important to note that sampling is somewhat simplified with liquid based cytology, which requires the use of a Cervex brush or similar sampling tool. Cervical smears are best performed at mid-cycle but the opportunity should not be missed to take a smear at other times, except during menstruation.

(3) A large number of women think that the main objective of cervical cytology is to detect cervical cancer and there are

probably an appreciable number who are deterred from having cervical smears because of this. The misconception is reinforced by using the term "cancer smear" and by telling women with negative smears that there was "no evidence of cancer/malignancy." When a subsequent smear shows "slight abnormalities" very reasonably the thought of cancer will come to mind and generate a great deal of unnecessary anxiety. Our health education message needs to change to ensure that women fully understand the purpose of cervical smears, that is to detect changes in the cells of the cervix which may, in a small number of cases, progress to cancer over many years. Greater emphasis should be made of the likelihood of minor abnormalities returning to normal and of the fact that if these minor changes persist or progress then treatment can be initiated and so prevent the development of cancer at a later date. Unfortunately, because there is currently no way of determining which changes will return to normal and which will progress, a number of women undergo unnecessary treatment. Continued surveillance of minor cervical pathology by cytology and colposcopy does cause anxiety and many women therefore prefer to opt for treatment.

11.2 SMEAR REPORT: TERMINOLOGY BRIEFLY EXPLAINED

Cervical smear terminology is rather complicated and can be very difficult to explain in simple lay terms. It is well worthwhile spending a little time discussing the possible results and their significance with the patient at the time of taking the smear and providing an information leaflet to take away. This may help to reduce anxiety should the smear need repeating at an earlier time interval or should there be a need to refer on for colposcopy.

11.2.1 Inadequate Specimen

There are a number of reasons why a smear is considered inadequate for assessment and some of these may be rectified before the smear is taken or sent to the laboratory.

(1) *Scanty specimen*. As mentioned above, if there is little material on the slide, repeat the sampling with a Cytobrush or Cervex brush. This should be mentioned on the smear form.
(2) *Blood stained specimen: too many red blood cells for adequate assessment*. Some cervices bleed profusely as the smear is taken. This may indicate cervicitis or too firm a pressure when

sampling. If there is some cervical mucus on the slide, it is probably worthwhile sending the specimen to the laboratory. If the smear appears to be purely blood, repeat at a later date. If bleeding occurs again then check for cervical infection, in particular *Chlamydia*. Consider treating with a tetracycline or alternatively refer to GU medicine for assessment.

(3) *Excessive bacteria*. This is usually due to bacterial vaginosis, a condition caused by an overgrowth of various bacteria, in particular *Gardnerella vaginalis*, *Mycoplasma hominis*, *Bacteroides* spp., and other anaerobes (see chapter 4). If these cover the specimen, the cervical cells are obscured and therefore cannot be properly assessed. Bacterial vaginosis usually requires treatment only if there are symptoms of vaginal discharge; however, when the condition interferes with cervical cytology consider treating before resampling.

(4) *Excess pus cells/polymorphs*. This may result from cervicitis or vaginitis. If you think clinically there is a vaginitis, take a swab for *Trichomonas* and *Candida* culture and treat with an antifungal. If there is clinical evidence of cervicitis, and this may be very difficult to assess, check for cervical pathogens such as *Chlamydia* and *N. gonorrhoeae*. Ideally, patients with presumed cervicitis should be referred to GU medicine for assessment.

    Candida may be seen on a cervical smear but it usually interferes with assessment only if there are excessive numbers of pus cells or candidal pseudohyphae and spores. Treatment is necessary only if symptoms are present or if the smear cannot be adequately assessed.

    Trichomonas vaginalis may also be seen on a cervical smear; however, it is always worth confirming with vaginal culture as false positive results may occur with cytology.

(5) *No endocervical component present*. There is continuing debate as to whether an adequate smear needs to contain endocervical and/or metaplastic cells. In fact, the only smears that can be judged with certainty as adequate are those containing abnormal cells. The presence of endocervical/metaplastic cells suggests that the squamo-columnar junction has been sampled, either partly or fully. If no endocervical component is present in a woman's first smear, consider repeating in 3 months. If previous smears have been negative, consider repeating in 1 year.

(6) *Poor spreading of material or poor fixation*. Always remember to spread the sample as evenly as possible over the slide and fix immediately before it air dries.

11.2.2 Inflammatory Smear

This is less commonly referred to nowadays; however, some cytology laboratories use this term to mean excessive pus cells suggesting inflammation and possible infection. More commonly, however, it refers to nuclear abnormalities insufficient to be termed dyskaryosis. If there is clinical evidence of cervicitis or the patient has noticed an increased discharge, either check for infection (*Chlamydia* and gonorrhea) in the surgery or preferably refer to GU medicine. If the cervix looks normal, repeat the smear in 3–6 months time. The inflammatory changes often resolve without antibiotic treatment. If inflammatory changes persist, check for infection as mentioned above and consider prescribing a course of tetracycline or erythromycin. If no infective cause is found and there is no improvement with antibiotics, refer for colposcopy.

11.2.3 Human Papillomavirus Infection (see also Chapter 18)

Human papillomavirus is the commonest sexually transmitted viral infection in the developed world. Although HPV causes genital warts, most HPV infection is "subclinical." Studies using extremely sensitive methods for detecting viral DNA (nucleic acid amplification test, such as polymerase chain reaction) have identified low levels of HPV in many sexually active women. This may either clear with time or persist indefinitely. Subclinical HPV infection can sometimes be diagnosed on cervical cytology by identifying cells called "koilocytes." The cells have a prominent nucleus and the cytoplasm contains a large perinuclear halo. These appearances are considered pathognomonic of HPV infection. Certain HPV types, in particular types 16 and 18, are strongly associated with high grade cervical dysplasia (cervical intraepithelial neoplasia (CIN) II/III) and neoplasia. For this reason, women with evidence of HPV on cervical cytology require careful follow-up and the usual recommendation is to repeat the smear after 6 months.

11.2.4 Borderline Nuclear Changes

This suggests nuclear abnormalities that are insufficient to be termed dyskaryosis. Borderline nuclear changes may be found in the presence of HPV infection, in association with inflammatory changes or in women with an IUCD. A borderline smear should be repeated in 6 months; if borderline changes persist, refer for colposcopy.

11.2.5 Dyskaryosis

This means that the cell nucleus is abnormal. There are three grades of dyskaryosis: mild, moderate, and severe. The equivalent histological terms are mild, moderate, and severe dysplasia or CIN I, II, and III. The concept of dyskaryosis is very difficult to explain in lay terms. The term "pre-cancer," although theoretically correct, is a little too dramatic and often causes anxiety. An "abnormality of the cells which is not cancerous but which may in a small number of women progress to cancer over many years" is rather wordy but fairly accurate and with emphasis on "not," "may," "small," and "many" tends to avoid leaving the patient with a feeling of pending doom. It can of course be difficult to achieve the right balance between causing undue anxiety and producing excessive complacency. Tailoring the wording to the individual patient is essential.

Women with smears showing moderate or severe dyskaryosis should be referred immediately for colposcopy. There is still debate as to whether women with mild dyskaryosis require immediate colposcopy or whether the smear should be repeated at 6 months and colposcopy reserved for women with persisting abnormalities. Although the evidence for immediate colposcopy is highly persuasive, such a policy would have important practical and financial implications. One must therefore be guided by local guidelines.

In the United States, smears showing evidence of HPV infection, borderline changes or mild dyskaryosis are grouped as *low-grade squamous epithelial lesions* (LGSIL). Moderate and severe dyskaryosis are grouped into *highgrade squamous epithelial lesions* (HGSIL). The term *atypical squamous cells of uncertain significance* (ASCUS) is used for cells considered abnormal but neither clearly reactive nor dysplastic. The above classification, known as the "Bethesda system," has generated some controversy, in particular with respect to the merging of HPV infection with mild dyskaryosis.

11.3 COLPOSCOPY

A number of studies have reported high levels of anxiety among women attending colposcopy clinics. Providing accurate information and carefully explaining how colposcopy is performed and what is likely to happen undoubtedly reduces the anxiety. Most women will be referred for colposcopy if mild cytological abnormalities persist (e.g. borderline changes or mild dyskaryosis) or if there is a single smear showing moderate or severe dyskaryosis. The following points should be covered at the time of referral.

(1) Explain that the colposcope is purely a magnifying system that enables the cervix to be examined in greater detail. It is

worth emphasizing that the colposcope does not enter the vagina and the procedure is rather like having a cervical smear. A weak vinegar solution (usually 5% acetic acid) is used to help show up abnormal areas on the cervix and this does very occasionally sting a little.

(2) If an abnormality is seen, a biopsy will be taken, usually without local anesthesia. Some women feel a short sharp pain as the biopsy is taken while others find this only mildly uncomfortable, likening the sensation to a firm pinch. A few colposcopists inject a small amount of local anesthetic prior to biopsy. This is very slightly uncomfortable but does ensure that the rest of the procedure is virtually painless.

(3) After a biopsy has been taken some women experience period-like pains that may persist for several hours. This is usually relieved by paracetamol or ibuprofen.

(4) There may be spotting of blood for a couple of days after taking a biopsy. Sexual intercourse should be avoided for a few days until healing occurs.

(5) The patient is usually asked to return in a couple of weeks for the result of histology and further management is discussed at that time. Some colposcopists prefer to "see and treat" on the first clinic attendance which usually involves performing a LLETZ.

(6) Most colposcopy clinics provide information leaflets for patients, which are sent out with the appointment. Providing information in the GP surgery at the time of referral is probably more appropriate and is best approached by having your local colposcopy clinic send details of their current management policy.

In the UK, colposcopy is recommended for the following groups:

- Three consecutive inadequate smears
- Three consecutive smears showing borderline nuclear changes in squamous cells
- One smear showing borderline nuclear changes in endocervical (glandular) cells
- Three smears reported as abnormal at any grade over a 10-year period
- Two consecutive smears showing mild dyskaryosis
- One smear showing moderate or severe dyskaryosis

11.3.1 Treatment of Cervical Intraepithelial Neoplasia

Although this will vary from unit to unit, LLETZ is the usual method used for treating CIN. This is usually performed under local anesthesia and has been shown to be a safe and effective procedure with no subsequent effect on menstruation or fertility. Repeat colposcopy is usually recommended 1 year after treatment and annual smears for 5 years.

Chapter 12

Contraception and Genital Tract Infection

Many GPs provide contraceptive advice to youngsters who have recently become sexually active or who are considering starting sexual relationships. In the UK, the median age of first sexual intercourse is 17 years for women aged 25–44 years and 16 for women aged 16–24 years. For men, this is 17 years for those aged between 20 and 44 years and 16 for those aged between 16 and 19. Over the last 10 years there has been an increase in the proportion of women having intercourse before the age of 16 years, whereas the proportion of men having intercourse before 16 has remained fairly constant for all ages. For 16–19 year olds, just under a third of men and a quarter of women report having had intercourse before the age of 16. The time between first sexual experience and first intercourse is 4 years for men and 3 years for women (i.e. age of first sexual experience is 13 years for men and 14 years for women). A number of studies have documented an association between early age at first intercourse and early menarche, early school leaving age, family disruption, and poor educational attainment. A recent large behavioral study in the UK found that just under a third of sexually active young women who left school at age 16 years with no qualifications had a child at age 17 years or younger. Young people who leave school later and with qualifications are less likely to have early intercourse, more likely to use contraception at first sex, be sexually competent and less likely to become pregnant.

Reassuringly, there has been an increase in condom use in the UK over the past 10 years with approximately three quarters of men and women reporting using a condom at first intercourse. There has also been a decrease in those using no contraception at first intercourse (approximately 10% of men and women under the age of 24 years). The UK has one of the highest teenage conception rates in Western Europe, with just over one-half of pregnancies in under 16-year-olds ending in termination.

These data emphasize the importance of providing the young and sexually active with easy access to contraception. The opportunity should also be taken to discuss other sexual health matters, in particular how to avoid acquiring sexually transmitted infections. This chapter looks at the issue of contraception and STIs in a little more detail.

12.1 CONDOMS

Laboratory studies have shown that latex condoms are effective mechanical barriers against hepatitis B virus, HIV, cytomegalovirus, herpes simplex virus, and *Chlamydia*.

Epidemiological studies have shown that correct and consistent use of condoms protect against gonorrhea, NGU, and HIV infection. There are conflicting data regarding protection from HPV infection, however, consistent condom use appears to offer some protection against genital warts, high grde CIN and cervical cancer and has also been found to produce higher rates of cervical HPV clearance and CIN regression. To be protective the condom must cover that part of the genital tract which is infected or likely to become infected, for example the cervix in the female and the urethra in the male. Protection is less likely for infections that may affect the vulva and perineum or the epithelium beyond the penile shaft, for example genital herpes and HPV infection.

There are a few points worth emphasizing. First, condoms must be used correctly, that is placed on to the penis before genital contact and unrolled fully to cover as much of the penis as possible. Teated condoms should have the air squeezed from the end as they are unrolled. Many youngsters do not know how to use a condom, particularly when they are being used for the first time. Condom manufacturers are usually happy to provide plastic demonstration models. These should be considered essential equipment for all GP surgeries and clinics that provide contraceptive or sexual health advice.

Condoms do occasionally split or slip off the penis during intercourse. Individuals who are particularly prone to these mishaps should check that they are fully unrolling the condom and that fingernails are not damaging the latex. In addition, some non-water-based lubricants and various vaginal preparations may damage latex and therefore should not be used in conjunction with either the condom or the diaphragm. The preparations include baby oil, petroleum jelly, Vaseline, 2% clindamycin cream, Ecostatin, Fungilin, Gyno-Daktarin, Gyno-Pevaryl, Monistat, Nizoral, Nystatin cream, Ortho Dienoestrol, Ortho Gynest, Premarin,

Sultrin, Witepsol-based suppositories, hair conditioner, skin softener, bath oil, massage oil, body oil, suntan oil, lipstick, cooking oil, margarine, butter, salad cream, cream, and ice cream!

A tremendous effort has been put into condom marketing in recent years and the larger manufacturers now provide a wide range of shapes, colors, and flavors. Apparently mint and Pina Colada flavored condoms are particularly well accepted. Occasionally low standard condoms find their way on to the market and for this reason, in the UK, only brands which display the British Standards "Kite Mark" should be used.

A common reason given by men for not using condoms is decreased sensitivity and hence reduced sexual pleasure. A technique termed "gel charging" does appear to heighten the sexual experience for some men and therefore may help to encourage condom use. This involves placing a small amount (e.g. a teaspoonful) of lubricant or spermicidal gel into the end of a condom before placing onto the penis. Contoured and flared condoms apparently give the most effective results.

12.2 DIAPHRAGM

Less information is available regarding the diaphragm, but the small number of studies which have been performed do show that this form of contraception provides women with protection against gonorrhea and other cervical infections.

Diaphragm use does appear to increase the risk of urinary tract infection.

12.3 SPERMICIDES

Nonoxynol-9 is a commonly used spermicide that also inhibits the growth of several sexually transmitted organisms. These include *N. gonorrhoeae*, *C. trachomatis*, *T. pallidum*, herpes simplex virus, cytomegalovirus, and HIV. It appears to have no action against HPV. Although many condoms are impregnated with spermicide, it is uncertain whether the amount present would be sufficient to kill these pathogens if the condom splits. There is also some concern that frequent use of nonoxynol-9 may produce vulvovaginal inflammation and possibly ulceration. These adverse reactions are of relevance to women having intercourse several times a day and are probably not applicable to the general sexually active population. Epidemiological studies on the use of spermicides have documented a protective effect against gonorrhea, trichomoniasis, and possibly *Chlamydia* and HIV. There appears to be no effect on bacterial vaginosis or candidiasis.

12.4 THE "FEMALE CONDOM"

The female condom, known in the UK as Femidom, is made from polyurethane. It has been shown in the laboratory to act as a complete barrier to cytomegalovirus, HIV, and to bacteriophages smaller than HIV and hepatitis B. The vaginal flora remains unchanged after repeated use and there is no evidence of an irritant effect on the vagina. A pregnancy rate of 2.6% during 6 months' use has been reported for "perfect users." Femidom is not acceptable to all women. It can be difficult to insert and occasionally the device can be pushed into the vagina or slip out. Hopefully, design modification will eventually resolve these problems. Unlike most male condoms, the lubricant on female condoms does not contain a spermicide.

12.5 INTRAUTERINE CONTRACEPTIVE DEVICE

The risk of PID among IUCD users has been generally overstated. There is a transient risk of developing infection at the time of or just after insertion that may be partly related to the degree of experience of the clinician fitting the device. PID affecting a women with an IUCD is often more severe clinically. Some studies have suggested a reduced risk of pelvic inflammatory disease amongst levonorgestrel-IUCD users compared with women using copper releasing devices.

12.6 HORMONAL CONTRACEPTIVES

Hormonal contraceptives have been shown to protect against PID and may reduce the degree of tubal inflammation if infection develops. Although some earlier studies did show an association between oral contraceptive use and chlamydial cervicitis, this has not been confirmed by more recent work. The use of injectable depot-medroxyprogesterone acetate has been reported to increase the risk of acquiring cervical chlamydial and gonococcal infection, possibly as a result of local immune suppression or by hormonally induced bacterial growth and persistence.

Chlamydia appears to be more frequently isolated from women with cervical ectopy, irrespective of the method of contraception used, probably owing to the organism preferentially infecting columnar epithelium rather than squamous epithelium.

12.7 IMPORTANT POINTS

(1) An ideal approach to contraception for the woman who is not in a steady relationship, or who may frequently change sexual partners, or who cannot guarantee the fidelity of her partner is to consider using both condoms and hormonal contraception.

The favored method of hormonal contraception is usually the oral contraceptive pill or a long acting reversible contraceptive. This approach provides optimal protection against STIs and pregnancy.

(2) All women starting oral or barrier contraception should receive information on emergency postcoital contraception. In particular, they need to know where emergency contraception is available and understand that it is appropriate to use "pills" up to 3 days and an IUCD up to 5 days after unprotected intercourse, although this may be extended and for IUCD use depends upon the time of ovulation. The term "morning after pill" gives the wrong message and should no longer be used. If unprotected intercourse was with a "new" partner, the possibility of acquiring a sexually transmitted infection should be discussed and referral to GU medicine advised. Women with a clinical suspicion or at risk for genital infection should ideally be screened for, in particular, *Chlamydia*, gonorrhea, and bacterial vaginosis and receive a course of tetracycline and metronidazole or co-amoxiclav prior to emergency IUCD insertion. Liaison with colleagues in GU medicine is to be recommended.

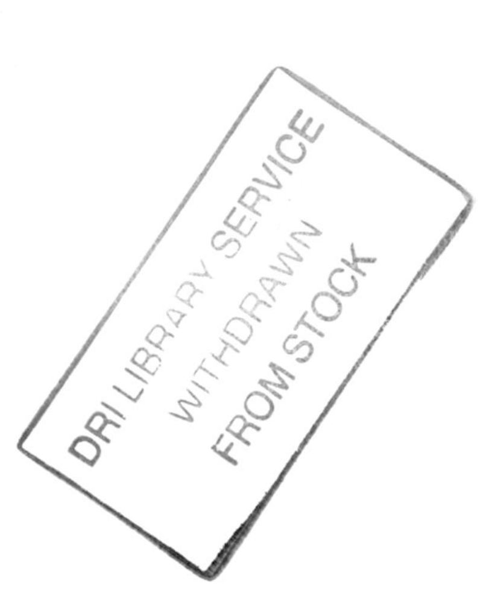
DRI LIBRARY SERVICE
WITHDRAWN
FROM STOCK

Chapter 13
Dysuria in Young Men

The commonest cause of dysuria in the young, single, sexually active male is urethritis rather than cystitis.

Urethritis is usually the result of a sexually acquired infection and may be conveniently divided into gonorrhea or "gonococcal urethritis" and "not-gonorrhea" or "non-gonococcal urethritis" (NGU). NGU is also known as "non-specific urethritis" (NSU).

Other symptoms associated with urethritis include urethral discharge, which may not be noticed by the patient, and frequency (Figure 13.1).

The following are the causes of NGU:

- *C. trachomatis* (40–60%). Although these cases should be called "chlamydial urethritis," the term "*Chlamydia*-positive NGU" is often used.
- *Mycoplasma genitalium*
- *Ureaplasma urealyticum* (? 10–20%). There is still some debate concerning the role of ureaplasmas in urethritis.

The following make up only a small percentage of cases, hence most NGU is truly non-specific, that is no specific organism can be isolated.

- *Trichomonas vaginalis*
- Herpes simplex virus
- Adenovirus (usually acquired through oral sex)
- *E. coli* (usually causes cystitis although it has been documented as a cause of urethritis in homosexual men)
- adenovirus (acquired by oral sex from a partner with adenovirus pharyngeal infection
- Certain anaerobes (e.g. *Bacteroides urealyticus*)
- Traumatic (e.g. postcatheterization, after pencil or biro insertion)
- Reactive (e.g. postdysenteric Reiter's syndrome may be associated with a urethritis). This is not sexually acquired.

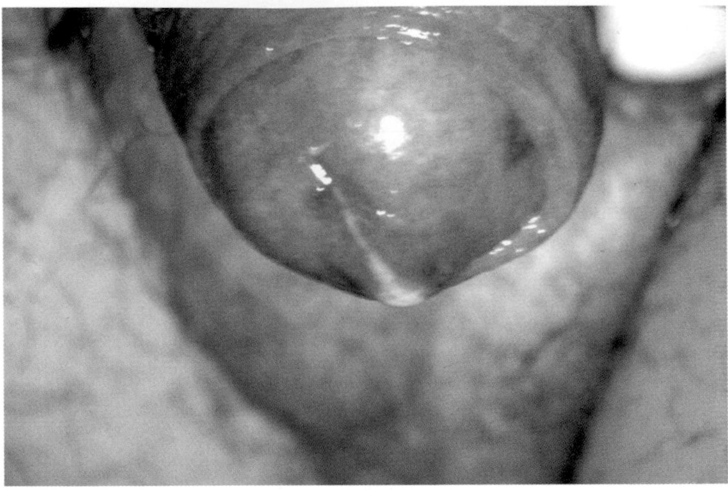

FIGURE 13.1. Mucoid urethral discharge due to chlamydia

13.1 INVESTIGATIONS

To diagnose urethritis the following investigations should be performed:

(1) *Urethral swab Gram stain*: A small foam swab or plastic loop is inserted into the opened meatus and the distal urethra gently swabbed. Secretions are then transferred on to a microscope slide for Gram staining and microscopy.

The presence of >4 polymorphs per HPF (×1000) is diagnostic of urethritis.

(2) *Two-glass urine test*: The patient is asked to pass the first 20–50 ml of his urinary stream into a glass and the second part of the stream into a second glass (any remaining in the bladder can be directed into the urinal). The presence of "threads" or "specks" of pus in the first glass with a clear second glass indicates an anterior urethritis. Pus in both glasses suggests a posterior urethritis or cystitis. If this is the case, send the first glass or an MSU to the laboratory for culture. Patients with a profuse discharge due to NGU or gonorrhea may show pus in both glasses; however, this will be much heavier in the first glass.

Phosphaturia is a common cause of cloudy urine and may be mistaken for pyuria. The addition of acetic acid will rapidly clear the urine if phosphates are present; if the urine remains cloudy then pyuria is the likely cause.

A rather more scientific method of diagnosing urethritis from the first catch urine is to examine the resuspended urinary sediment under the microscope. The presence of >15 polymorphs in any of five random fields (×400) indicates a urethritis. Some studies have suggested that examination of the urine may be a more sensitive method of detecting mild urethritis than the urethral Gram stain.

Cases of mild urethritis may be missed if the patient has recently passed urine before the above investigations are performed. For this reason, patients should be asked to hold on to their urine for at least three hours prior to assessment. If the history is suggestive of urethritis and the initial investigations prove negative, repeat testing should be performed early in the morning, the patient having held on to his urine overnight.

(3) Whenever possible, a urethral swab should also be taken for detection of *Chlamydia*, as occasionally chlamydial infection may be present in the absence of an obvious urethritis. Finding *Chlamydia*, however, does not alter patient management. Tetracycline is first-line treatment for both *Chlamydia*-positive and *Chlamydia*-negative NGU.

(4) Gonococcal urethritis is far less common than NGU, but a urethral swab should be taken for *N. gonorrhoeae* culture. Remember that the gonococcus is particularly delicate and may well not survive an overnight delay before plating on to specific culture media. If there is likely to be a delay, place the swab in the refrigerator rather than keeping at room temperature. However, if gonorrhea is considered a possible diagnosis, the patient should ideally be referred to GU medicine so that swabs may be plated on to the appropriate culture media and incubated prior to transport to the laboratory. The important issue of contact tracing can also be addressed.

(5) Most laboratories are currently unable to routinely test for *Mycoplasma genitalium* infection.

(6) Send an MSU or first-catch urine for microscopy and culture if the two-glass urine test suggests posterior urethritis/cystitis of urine dipstix testing shows the presence of nitrites or blood.

13.2 MANAGEMENT OF NON-GONOCOCCAL URETHRITIS

Most GP surgeries do not have access to immediate microscopy and there may be a delay in transporting microbiology specimens to the laboratory; therefore, patients with suspected urethritis should be referred to GU medicine for assessment. Urethritis is considered an urgent problem requiring immediate attention. A telephone call to the clinic before sending along the patient is appreciated, however, as most clinics run an appointment system.

First-line treatment for NGU should be with either a tetracycline or azithromycin. Oxytetracycline 500 mg qds for 10 days is relatively cheap but compliance may be poor compared with, for example, doxycycline 100 mg bd for 7days.
Azithromycin 1 g stat or 500 mg stat followed by 250 mg daily for four days are useful alternatives, both providing good coverage for chlamydial infection with the five day course being more effective against *Mycoplasma genitalium* infection.

Erythromycin stearate 500 mg bd for 14 days and ofloxacin 200 mg bd for 7 days are alternative second-line treatment options.

Sexual partners must be assessed and an antibiotic prescribed, namely a tetracycline, azithromycin or erythromycin, even in the absence of infection. The possibility of missing a chlamydial infection with the subsequent development of asymptomatic pelvic infection leading to infertility or ectopic pregnancy warrants such a policy.

Patients should be reassessed following treatment to ensure cure. Resolution of symptoms does not always indicate eradication of infection, hence the importance of repeating tests after treatment. The initial lack of response to treatment may result from poor compliance, reinfection, or persistent infection. If persistence is considered likely, retreat with erythromycin or azithromycin (or tetracycline if erythromycin or azithromycin was used as first-line treatment). Reinforce the need to avoid sexual intercourse until partners have been assessed and treated and advise against frequent self-examination, masturbation, spicy foods, and excessive alcohol that may aggravate symptoms. A longer course of tetracycline together with metronidazole should be considered if the urethritis persists. Patients with continued symptoms together with objective evidence of urethritis may warrant urethroscopy, urethral ultrasound, or a urethrogram.

13.2.1 Recurrent Urethritis

A small number of men suffer repeated episodes of NGU. Some of these will be caused by reinfection from new or previously untreated partners; however, recurrence of urethritis without sexual contact or within a relationship where the sexual partner has received treatment is well recognized. If both partners are monogamous, further treatment of the female partner is probably not warranted. Most clinicians would re-treat the symptomatic male although previous courses of tetracycline, azithromycin and erythromycin significantly reduce the likelihood of ongoing infection.

Some cases of recurrent urethritis are thought to be due to "immunological hypersensitivity" to a previous infection that results in a persisting inflammatory response.

13.3 MANAGEMENT OF GONORRHEA

Patients with gonorrhea should be referred to a GU medicine clinic for treatment, follow-up, and contact tracing (Figure 13.2). If there is a delay before the patient can be seen, consider treating with oral cefixime 400 mg or cefrtriaxone 250 mg i.m. and then refer to the GU medicine clinic for follow-up and contact tracing.

Penicillin and ciprofloxacin resistant gonorrhea is now seen in the UK, hence the move to using a cephalosporin. Most laboratories will provide details of antibiotic sensitivities for their gonococcal isolates.

Prescribing a 7-day course of tetracycline in addition to anti-gonococcal treatment to cover possible coinfection with *Chlamydia* is to be recommended. Patients should reattend for "tests of cure" after treatment and to follow up issues regarding partner notification.

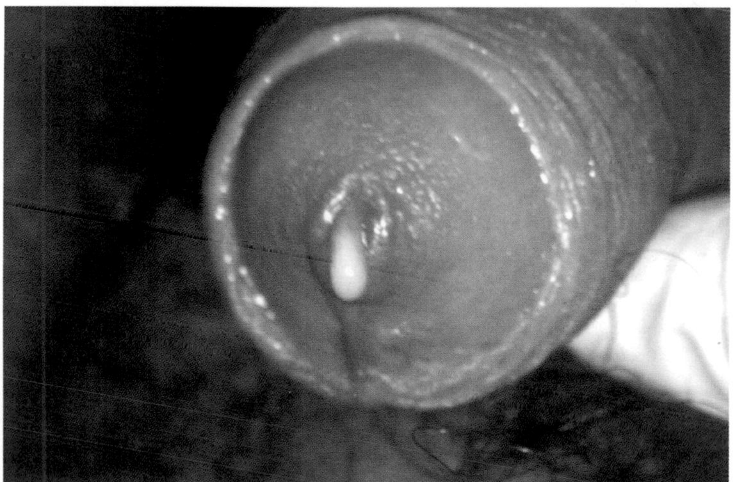

Figure 13.2. Mucopurulent urethral discharge due to gonorrhoea

13.4 MANAGEMENT OF URINARY TRACT INFECTION

As mentioned above, dysuria in the young, sexually active male is more likely to be due to urethritis than to cystitis or urinary tract infection. If a UTI is considered the most likely diagnosis, consider treating with antibiotics which achieve therapeutic concentrations in the prostate (e.g. trimethoprim, norfloxacin, ciprofloxacin).

Men with acute pyelonephritis or who suffer more than one episode of cystitis warrant urological investigation.

13.5 IMPORTANT POINTS

(1) Consider a diagnosis of urethritis rather than cystitis in the "unmarried," sexually active man with dysuria. Urethritis should also be considered in the married or cohabiting man but proceed with a little more caution!

(2) Initial investigations should include a urethral Gram stain and two-glass urine test. If both glasses of the two-glass urine test contain pus, send off the first glass or an MSU for microscopy and culture and treat as cystitis.

(3) If microscopy is unavailable in the GP surgery, the patient should be referred to a GU medicine clinic for urgent assessment. Contact tracing can then also be addressed and the opportunity taken to provide health education and information about the condition.

(4) Remember that "contact tracing" or "partner notification" involves rather more than providing antibiotics for the sexual partner. Partners should be clinically assessed and the possibility of other sexual partners being involved must be addressed.

(5) Consider the diagnosis of urethritis in men and women with dysuria and an MSU showing sterile pyuria.

(6) NGU is sexually acquired in the majority of cases. Sexual partners must be assessed and treated.

(7) Although this chapter has focused on men presenting with dysuria, remember that both gonococcal and, in particular, NGU may be asymptomatic. Such individuals may pass on their infection unknowingly to sexual partners and act as important transmitters of disease within the community.

Chapter 14

Prostatitis, Chronic Pelvic Pain Syndrome, and Hematospermia

Men with "prostatitis" often find their way to either urology or GU medicine.

Acute bacterial (Type I) prostatitis commonly presents with fever, chills, frequency, dysuria or strangury, and rectal pain. Examination reveals a tender, swollen prostate gland.

Chronic bacterial (Type II) prostatitis (CBP) may be more difficult to diagnose clinically. Symptoms may include perineal or suprapubic discomfort or pain sometimes radiating to the testes and penis. This may be associated with dysuria, frequency, and postejaculatory pain. CBP may also present as recurrent urinary tract infection. Rectal examination does not usually reveal prostatic tenderness. True CBP is thought to account for approximately 5% of cases of symptomatic prostatitis.

Chronic pelvic pain syndrome (CPPS) (Type III) accounts for the remaining 95% of cases and is subdivided into inflammatory (Type IIIa) (formerly known as "chronic abacterial prostatitis") and non-inflammatory (Type IIIb) (formerly known as "prostatodynia"). Type IIIa and IIIb are equally prevalent and may even be the same condition. Men with CPPS are usually young to middle-aged and present with perineal or genital pain lasting for several weeks or months. Pain is central to the diagnosis and is usually variable in intensity and typically widely distributed in the genital, perineal, and pelvic areas. There may be associated urinary symptoms such as frequency, variable urine flow, and urgency and sexual disturbance in the form of ejaculatory discomfort.

Other causes of "prostatitis-like" symptoms are as follows:

- Bladder neck dyssynergia (muscular incoordination) may present with frequency, urgency, and postmicturition dribbling. Diagnosis is usually by urinary flow studies.

- Pelvic floor tension myalgia presents with frequency, urgency, and perineal discomfort and there is pain on palpating the levator ani.
- Pudendal neuralgia may present with perineal and genital pain.
- Benign sacral meningeal cysts have been reported as a cause of genital pain and are best visualized by magnetic resonance imaging (MRI) scanning of the lumbosacral spine. However, it is probably prudent to consider seeking a neurological or urological opinion before embarking on costly investigations.

14.1 INVESTIGATIONS

Diagnosing chronic prostatitis can be difficult in general practice. "Localization studies" are no longer felt to be necessary as a similar percentage of normal controls have been found to have positive cultures of expressed prostatic secretions as CPPS patients.

Mid-stream urine culture should be performed as this may be positive in some patients with type II prostatitis.

Transrectal ultrasound should be necessary only if a prostatic abscess is suspected or as part of a research study.

14.2 TREATMENT

An urgent urological opinion should be sought for patients with presumed acute prostatitis. The condition is usually caused by the common urinary pathogens (e.g. *E. coli, Proteus* spp., *Streptococcus faecalis, Klebsiella* spp., *Pseudomonas* spp.) and is best treated with trimethoprim or a 4-quinolone such as ciprofloxacin or ofloxacin. Intravenous therapy is usually required initially and treatment should continue with oral antibiotics for up to 6 weeks.

Chronic bacterial prostatitis requires an antibiotic that can pass readily into the prostate. A 6–8-week course of ciprofloxacin (500 mg bd) or ofloxacin 400 mg daily should be considered. Trimethoprim is less effective in this condition.

Patients with CPPS often prove difficult to manage. The following have been reported as potentially useful.

- A 6-week course of antibiotics is often tried although their role in the management of CPPS is not well defined. Ofloxacin or ciprofloxacin are reasonable choices. Doxycycline (100 mg bd) has the possible advantage of an anti-inflammatory as well as an antibacterial action and may be tried if quinolones are ineffective.

- Non-steroidal anti-inflammatory drugs (NSAIDs) are sometimes given at the same time as antibiotics, either orally or, possibly preferably, as suppositories.
- Low to medium dose amitriptyline (e.g. 25–75 mg), as used for chronic pain control, may prove helpful and antidepressants (e.g. fluoxetine) if a co-existent depressive element is suspected.
- Some patients with CPPS have a spastic dysfunction of the bladder neck and prostatic urethra and may benefit from an alpha-blocker (e.g. tamsulosin, terazosin).
- Finasteride (5 mg daily) is worth trying if there is evidence of co-existent prostatic enlargement.
- The bioflavanoid, quercetin (500 mg bd for one month) may prove helpful if pain is the predominant feature rather than urinary symptoms.
- Pollen extract (cernilton) is reported to have anti-inflammatory and anti-adrenergic properties and has been used successfully in some cases of CPPS. Treatment may need to be continued for some months.
- Microwave hyperthermia to the prostate has also been used with variable success.
- Psychological factors should be tactfully sought and addressed and the use of acupuncture, hypnosis or relaxation, and visualization techniques considered. Most importantly, time should be taken to explain that the condition is not precancerous, will not affect fertility, and cannot be passed on or acquired through sexual intercourse.
- The natural history of CPPS is often fluctuating and symptoms may resolve over time.
- Referral to a chronic pain clinic should be considered in patients with persisting symptoms.

14.3 HEMATOSPERMIA

Blood in the ejaculate is a worrying condition that often raises concerns about cancer or sexually transmitted infection. It is important to distinguish a blood stained ejaculate from fresh bleeding per urethra (e.g. secondary to intrameatal or distal urethral warts) and traumatic lesions (e.g. a torn frenulum). A careful genital and prostatic examination are therefore required and the appropriate tests taken to check for urethritis, including chlamydial and gonococcal infection, although in the majority of cases these prove negative. The blood pressure should be measured and urinalysis performed to exclude hematuria.

Men over 40 years of age with no other urinary or genital symptoms require reassurance. The condition may recur but will eventually cease. Men over 45 years of age are at greater risk of having underlying pathology and should undergo further investigation, including prostate specific antigen (PSA) testing after appropriate counseling.

Chapter 15
Scrotal Pain

The scrotum and its contents have a complicated nerve supply.

(1) Sympathetic fibers from T1–L1 supply the testis, vas, and epididymis.
(2) Somatic fibers from L1–L2 supply the outer surface of the testis, the tunica vaginalis, and the anterior scrotal skin.
(3) Somatic fibers from S2–S3 supply the rest of the scrotal skin.

Scrotal pain may therefore be caused by intrascrotal pathology or result from referred pain from visceral or somatic structures.

Causes of referred pain include the following:

(1) Impacted stone in the lower ureter (splanchnic L1)
(2) Small inguinal hernia compressing the genitofemoral nerve
(3) Degenerative lesions of the lower thoracic and upper lumbar spine
(4) Tendonitis at the insertion of the inguinal ligament into the pubis
(5) Disease of the genital viscera (e.g. prostate, seminal vesicles)
(6) Benign sacral meningeal cysts (see also vulvodynia p. 45)
(7) Aneurysm of the internal iliac artery.

15.1 INTRASCROTAL PATHOLOGY

15.1.1 Epididymitis

The commonest cause of acute scrotal pain in the adult is acute epididymitis. In sexually active men under the age of about 35 years, this is usually caused by *C. trachomatis*. The patient presents with "pain in the scrotum," but there is often an associated urethritis, which may be asymptomatic. In men over the age of 35 years, the commonest causes of epididymitis are the more standard urinary tract pathogens such as *E. coli*, *Pseudomonas* spp., *Klebsiella* spp., and *Proteus* spp.

15.1.1.1 Investigations

The sexual history may give a clue as to whether the condition is more likely to be sexually or non-sexually transmitted.

In the younger, sexually active single male, the initial investigations should include the following (see also chapter 13-page 74):

- urethral swab for Gram stain (to look for evidence of urethritis)
- urethral swabs for detection of *Chlamydia* (urine test preferred by patient but not currently routinely available in the UK) and possibly gonorrhea culture
- two-glass urine test
- MSU or send off the first glass of the two-glass urine for culture.

In the "older" age groups, culture of an MSU may be sufficient.

15.1.1.2 Management

The "young" sexually active male with epididymitis should ideally be referred to a GU medicine clinic for urgent investigation. If evidence of urethritis is found or a sexually transmitted cause considered likely then treat with an antibiotic active against *Chlamydia*, such as a tetracycline (e.g. doxycycline 100 mg bd). The patient should be reviewed in 1 week or sooner if symptoms worsen. If there is clinical improvement, the treatment should be continued for at least 6 weeks. Sexual contacts must be assessed, in particular for evidence of chlamydial infection.

If a urinary tract pathogen is considered a more likely cause, treatment with, for example, trimethoprim, norfloxacin, or ofloxacin should be started while awaiting the results of MSU culture and sensitivity tests.

Many patients find a scrotal support helpful in addition to simple analgesia.

If there is any doubt about the diagnosis, an urgent urological opinion should be requested to exclude torsion of the testis.

15.1.2 Testicular (Spermatic Cord) Torsion

Just under 50% of men with testicular torsion give a history of previous brief episodes of scrotal discomfort. The pain is usually of sudden onset and severe. Torsion is more common in young men (late teens) and should be considered in this age group if tests for urethritis and upper urinary tract infection prove negative. All patients with a suspected torsion should be referred urgently for a urological opinion with the view to emergency exploration of the scrotum.

15.1.3 Orchitis

This may affect one or both testes and in the UK it is most commonly associated with mumps. Testicular atrophy develops in approximately 15% of adults following severe mumps orchitis. More unusual causes of orchitis include infectious mononucleosis, coxsackie B virus infection, and dengue fever.

15.1.4 Tumor

Approximately 10% of testicular tumors present as a painful swelling and may be initially misdiagnosed as epididymitis. More commonly, however, tumors are painless or may be detected as a firmness or asymmetry of the testis, sometimes associated with aching or discomfort. Ultrasound scanning helps distinguish between masses in the body of the testis and other intrascrotal swellings and should also be considered in patients with possible epididymo-orchitis that fails to resolve within a couple of weeks.

15.1.5 Peri-orchitis

This presents as a tender nodule on the surface of the testis and results from inflammation in the tunica vaginalis. Symptoms usually improve with time without the need for surgery.

15.1.6 Cremasteric Spasm

This may cause pain or discomfort, particularly during intercourse, and is associated with the testis being drawn up to the external inguinal ring. This may be relieved by circumcision of the cremaster which divides the genitofemoral nerve.

15.1.7 Epididymal Cysts

These are common and usually painless. Pain or discomfort may result from bleeding within a cyst. Referral is not required for asymptomatic cysts.

15.1.8 After Vasectomy

Scrotal discomfort after vasectomy may be caused by obstruction and distension of the epididymal duct. This is usually relieved by using a scrotal support and treatment with NSAIDs.

A small, tender swelling at the site of the vasectomy is frequently a sperm granuloma and may appear months or years after the procedure. If the pain fails to settle with a scrotal support and NSAIDs, a surgical excision or epididymectomy may be required.

15.1.9 Varicocele

Varicoceles may cause aching within the scrotum which becomes worse toward the end of the day. Thrombosis within a varicocele has been reported as a cause of scrotal pain.

15.1.10 Idiopathic

In many young men with scrotal pain, the only abnormality found is a rather sensitive epididymis. This may result from "seminal congestion" and is best treated by reassurance.

15.2 IMPORTANT MANAGEMENT POINTS

(1) Consider referral to GU medicine if you think there is evidence of epididymitis.
(2) Consider urgent referral to urology if there is a possibility of torsion.
(3) Scrotal ultrasound is a useful non-invasive procedure that may help to determine the nature of intrascrotal pathology. It may also help to reassure both patient and doctor that no serious pathology is present.

Chapter 16
Penile Rashes

Inflammation of the glans penis (balanitis) and of the prepuce (posthitis) usually occur together.

16.1 IRRITANT BALANOPOSTHITIS

Very common and usually the result of poor hygiene. An accumulation of smegma may be visible (Figure 16.1). Advise gentle bathing twice daily with plain or slightly salty water followed by application of a barrier cream (e.g. aqueous cream).

16.1.1 CANDIDIASIS

Usually presents as a diffuse erythema with numerous scattered small, red, slightly "eroded" spots (Figure 16.2), although an erosive balanitis has been reported.

16.1.2 BACTERIAL INFECTION

Anaerobic bacteria and group B streptococci occasionally cause a balanoposthitis (Figure 16.3). In the early stages of infection, gentle bathing followed by a barrier cream may be sufficient treatment.

16.1.3 DERMATITIS

Seborrheic dermatitis and contact dermatitis may present on the penis. Ask about other skin problems (e.g. affecting the scalp or face) and whether there is a history of allergy. Treat initially with hydrocortisone cream. If there is secondary infection, consider using a combined steroidal/antibacterial/antifungal preparation.

16.2 LESS COMMON CAUSES OF BALANOPOSTHITIS

16.2.1 Circinate Balanitis

Associated with Reiter's syndrome or, more frequently, with the incomplete syndrome (i.e. reactive arthritis with or without urethritis or conjunctivitis) (Figure 16.4).

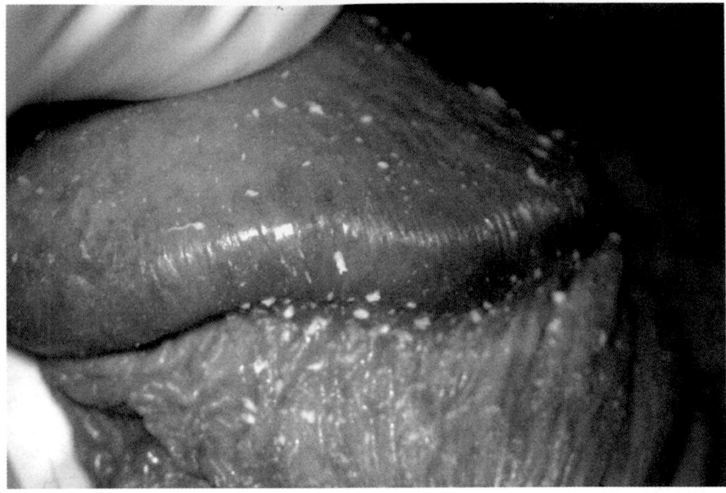

FIGURE 16.1. Irritant posthitis – smegma present

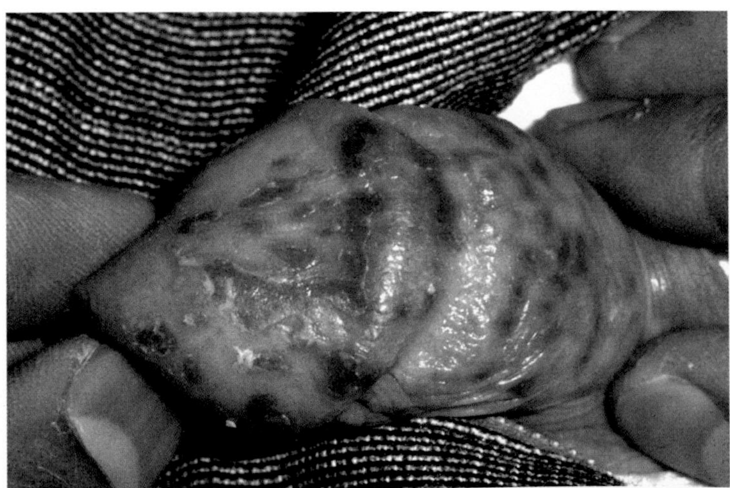

FIGURE 16.2. Penile candidiasis

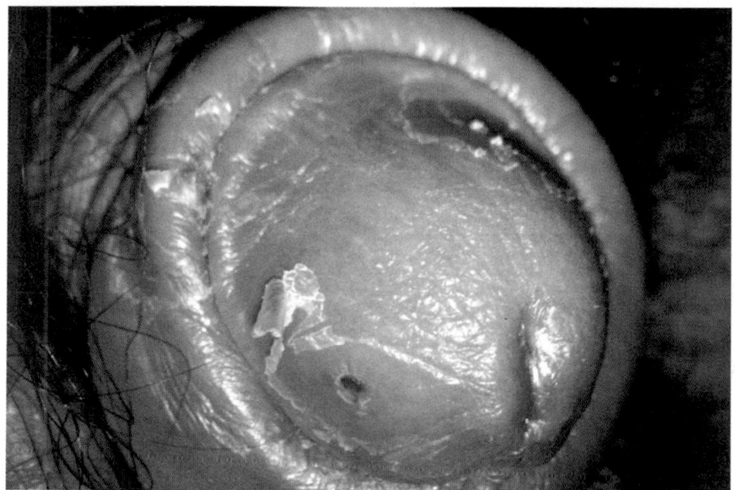

FIGURE 16.3. Streptococcal balanoposthitis

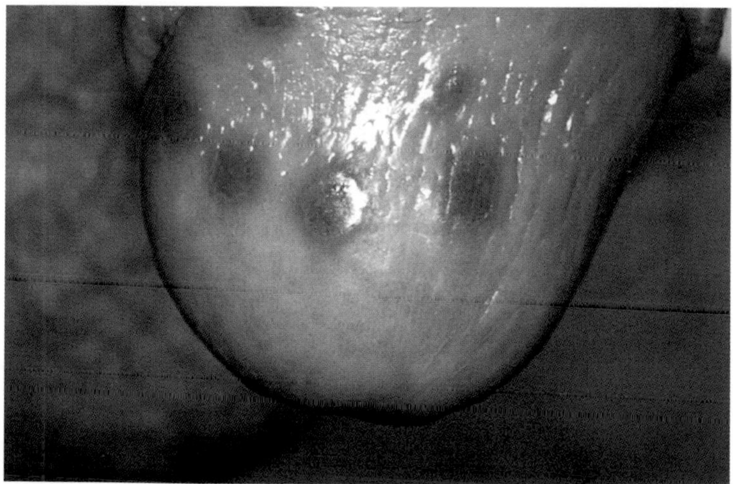

FIGURE 16.4. Circinate balanitis

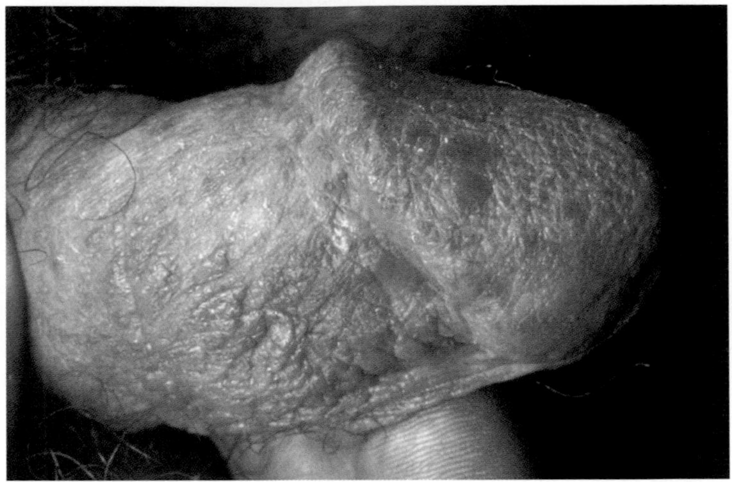

FIGURE 16.5. Lichen planus

16.2.2 Lichen Planus

Usually presents with well-demarcated red-purplish lesions and may be confused with flat warts or psoriasis (Figure 16.5).

16.2.3 Psoriasis

Genital lesions frequently lose the classical silvery scale and present as erythematous plaques (Figure 16.6).

16.2.4 Lichen Sclerosus

Areas of erythema with whitened, atrophic patches are the typical features (Figure 16.7). Adhesions may occur between the glans penis and the prepuce and long-standing cases may progress to phimosis. Perimeatal disease leads to narrowing of the urethral meatus (Figure 16.8). Treat initially with a potent topical steroid (e.g. clobetasol propionate) and then slowly "wean down" according to clinical response. Daily application for 4-weeks and then 2–3 times weekly for a further 2 months is a reasonable approach with review at 3 months. As some patients are hesitant to apply steroids to their genitalia, it is important to explain the importance of this treatment and provide reassurance that long-term application is safe under clinical supervision. Preputial tightening secondary to lichen sclerosus

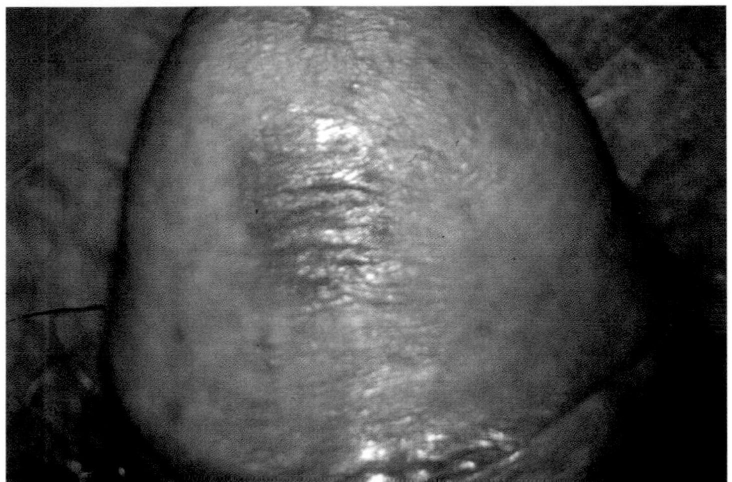

FIGURE 16.6. Psoriasis

can be dramatically improved with topical steroids and may obviate the need for circumcision. Long-term follow-up is recommended because of the small risk of developing squamous cell carcinoma.

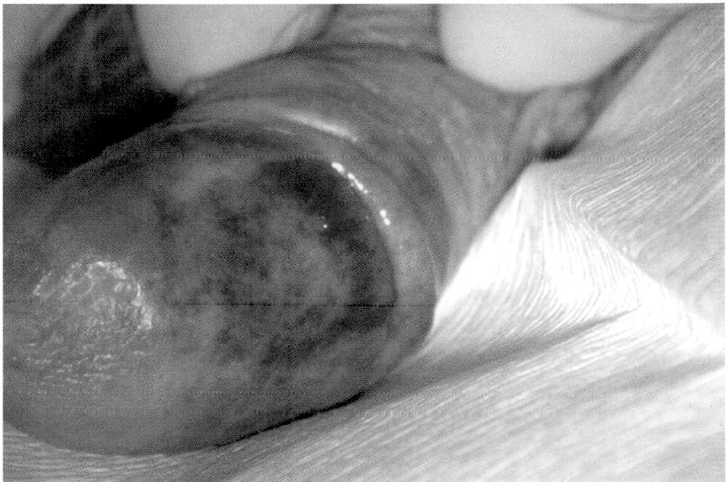

FIGURE 16.7. Lichen sclerosus – note early adhesions between the prepuce and glans

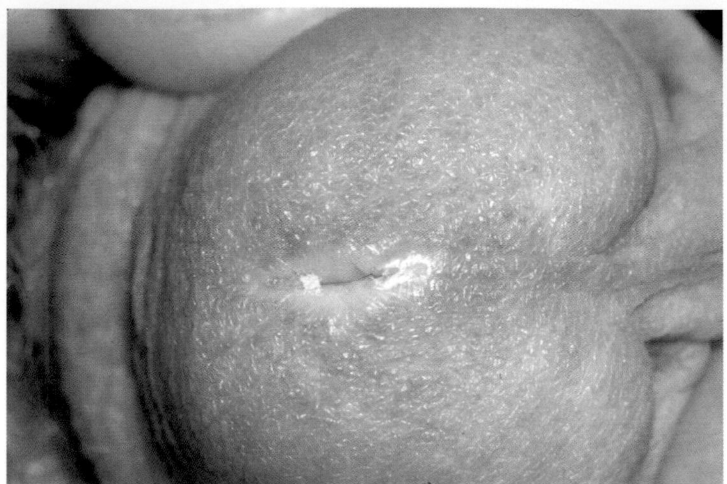

FIGURE 16.8. Lichen sclerosus – atrophic changes and narrowing of the meatus

16.2.5 Human Papillomavirus Infection

A patchy balanoposthitis may predate the appearance of classical condylomata acuminata (genital warts).

Penile intraepithelial neoplasia (frequently caused by HPV type 16) may present as mildly erythematous papules (Figure 16.9).

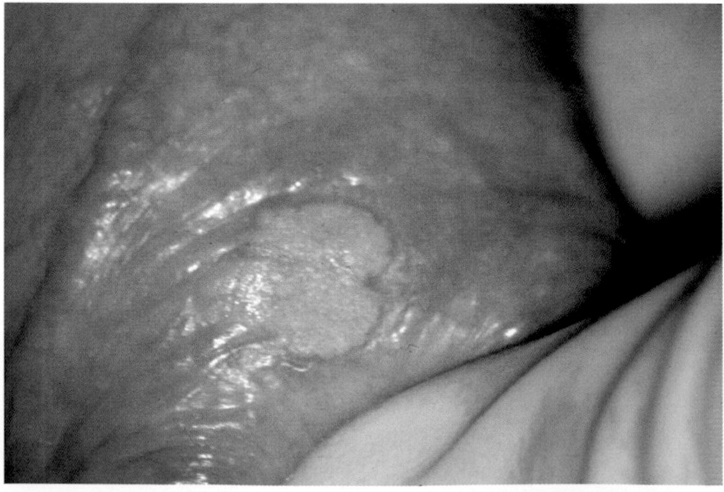

FIGURE 16.9. Penile intraepithelial neoplasia (PIN)

16.2.6 Fixed Drug Eruptions

Although many drugs have the potential to cause a fixed drug eruption, it is more commonly seen with tetracyclines, trimethoprim, sulphonamides, non-steroidal anti-inflammatories, paracetamol, and salicylates. Lesions may first appear as a patch of erythema or a small blister and can rapidly progress to produce large areas of ulceration (Figure 16.10). Secondary infection can occur and treatment should include gentle bathing with salty water and, in some cases, a mild anti-inflammatory plus antibacterial cream. Oral prednisolone is very occasionally required for the more severe and extensive cases.

16.2.7 Zoon's Balanitis (Plasma Cell Balanitis)

An uncommon condition seen mostly in middle-aged and elderly men. The lesions present as flat, moist, red, shiny plaques affecting the glans and mucosa of the prepuce (Figure 16.11). Irritation is common. Although circumcision is a recommended treatment, some cases do respond to aeration and topical moderate-strength steroids, particularly those preparations containing an antibacterial agent.

16.2.8 Erythroplasia of Queyrat

An uncommon condition now falling under the diagnostic category of "penile intraepithelial neoplasia" (PIN). Erythroplasia is

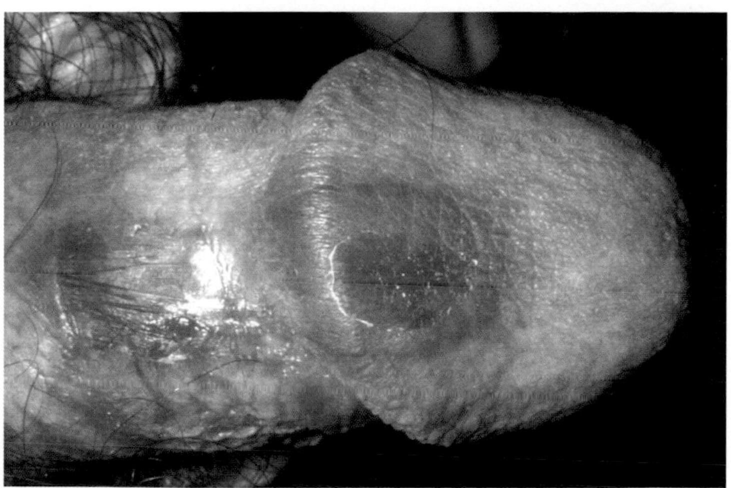

FIGURE 16.10. Fixed drug eruption

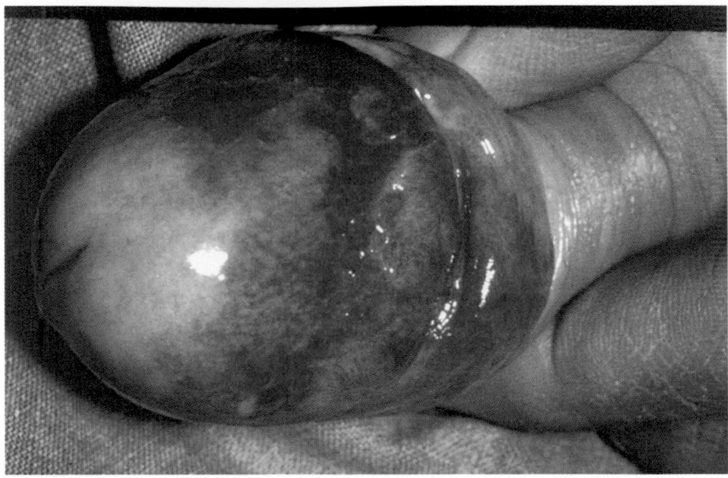

FIGURE 16.11. Zoon's balanitis

seen almost exclusively in uncircumcised men and lesions appear as well-demarcated shiny, red, velvety plaques. Malignant change is well documented.

16.2.9 Other Penile and Scrotal Rashes

16.2.9.1 Kaposi's Sarcoma

Kaposi's sarcoma is seen mostly in patients with HIV infection in the UK and is caused by human herpes virus type 8. Lesions are initially flat and dusky red and may appear on the glans penis or shaft.

16.2.9.2 Angiokeratomata

These small lesions usually affect the scrotum rather than the penis and appear as tiny, often multiple, bright red vascular spots. They may increase in number and size with age and are harmless.

16.2.9.3 Melanocytic Naevi

These may appear on the penis or scrotum and have the same characteristics as naevi elsewhere on the body.

16.3 GENERAL ADVICE FOR PATIENTS WITH BALANOPOSTHITIS

Aeration is helpful for most causes of balanitis but can sometimes be difficult to achieve. Keeping the foreskin retracted for an hour or so each evening and allowing a good circulation of air, perhaps under a dressing gown or nightshirt for social acceptability, is worth trying. A combined topical steroid and antibacterial cream, if indicated, can then be applied and the foreskin pulled back over the glans. It is unnecessary to use large amounts of cream and patients should be advised accordingly.

Gentle bathing with salty water is often soothing, particularly for moist lesions. The area can then be dried with a hair dryer on cool setting.

Chapter 17
Genital Ulceration

17.1 GENITAL HERPES

Herpes simplex virus (HSV) infection is by far the commonest cause of genital ulceration seen in general practice. Although HSV type 2 has traditionally been considered the commonest cause of genital herpes, studies have reported HSV type 1 infection in over 60% of cases, the virus being passed on by oro-genital contact.

Serological studies examining HSV-2 seroprevalence in various population groups have shown that up to 70% of infections are asymptomatic.

17.2 CLINICAL FEATURES

17.2.1 Primary attack (i.e. No previous exposure to HSV-1 or HSV-2)

Primary herpes is a miserable condition. Following an incubation period of 3–5 days (range 1–40 days), small blisters appear on the genitalia, often associated with a "flu-like" illness. The blisters soon break down to leave small tender ulcers that may eventually merge to produce quite extensive areas of painful ulceration (Figures 17.1 and 17.2). Lesions start to heal after about 12 days.

Herpes may cause a urethritis which presents as dysuria, often severe in nature.

Ninety percent of women have a cervicitis producing an excessive "vaginal" discharge.

Other clinical features include painful inguinal lymphadenopathy, headache and photophobia (aseptic meningitis), urinary retention (sacral radiculopathy), pharyngitis, and extragenital lesions (on fingers, lips, buttocks).

17.2.2 First Attack: Non-primary

This is the first clinical episode of herpes in a patient who has had previous exposure to the virus (type 1 or type 2). Symptoms are usually much less severe than primary herpes owing to partial immunity.

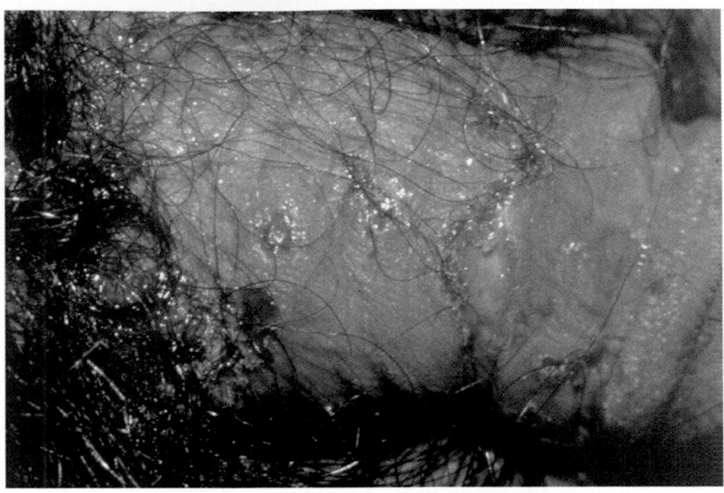

FIGURE 17.1. Primary genital herpes affecting the penis

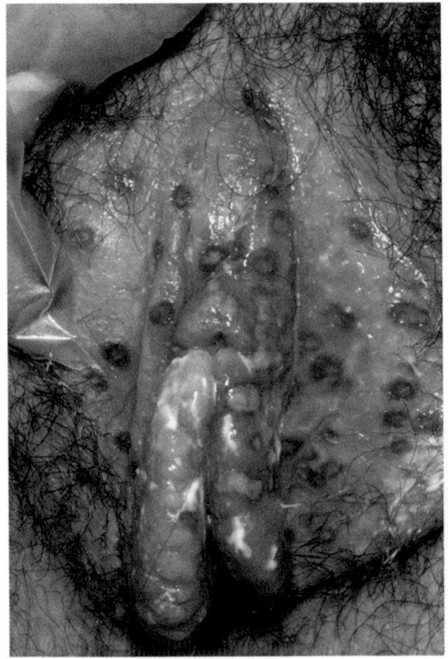

FIGURE 17.2. Primary genital herpes affecting the vulva

17.2.3 Recurrent Herpes

Approximately 90% of patients with type 2 genital herpes will suffer a recurrence within 1 year of their primary attack. This is in contrast to patients with HSV type 1 infection, in whom there is a 55% chance of recurrence. The frequency of recurrences also differs between the two viral types – on average 3–4 attacks per year with HSV-2 infection compared with twice a year with HSV-1.

Viral reactivation leading to symptomatic or asymptomatic viral shedding may be greatest during the first few months after a primary attack and should be discussed with patients diagnosed with primary infection. Symptoms of recurrent genital herpes are often mild. About 50% of patients will develop prodromal symptoms such as genital "pins and needles," shooting pains in the buttocks and legs, or inguinal discomfort associated with lymphadenopathy. Symptoms of sacral neuralgia are the most troublesome part of the recurrence for some patients.

The cervix is affected in only 10% of women with recurrent disease.

When lesions appear they tend to be few in number and heal within 1 week. A small number of patients, however, suffer more frequent and long-lasting attacks that can be particularly distressing (Figures 17.3 and 17.4).

Recent studies have suggested that symptoms of recurrent disease may be minimal and often ignored by the patient. This is an important issue that should be addressed when the diagnosis

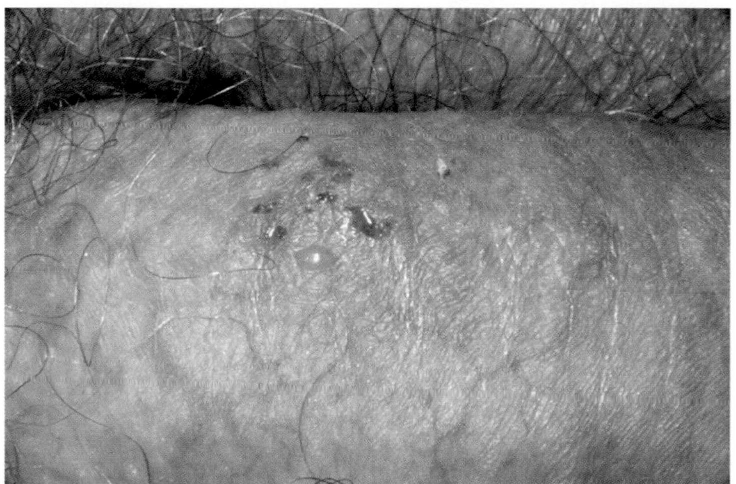

FIGURE 17.3. Recurrent herpes of the penis

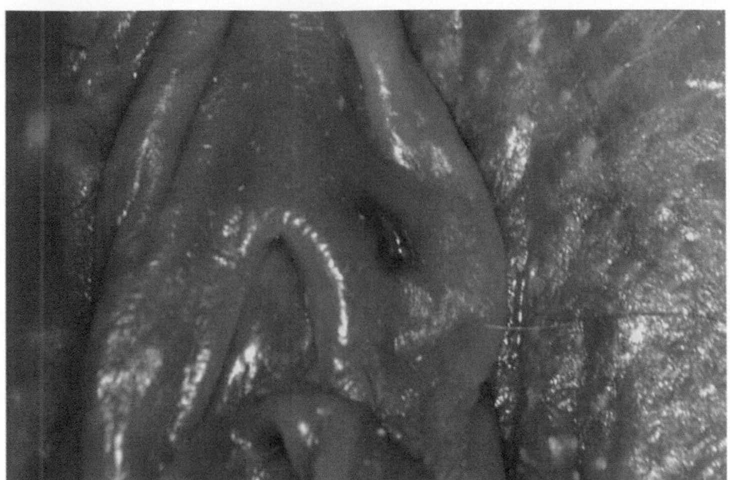

FIGURE 17.4. Recurrent herpes of the vulva

of herpes is first made. Taking note of minor genital symptoms and avoiding sexual contact at such times is important if the risk of transmission to partners is to be reduced.

It is always wise to confirm the clinical diagnosis of herpes by positive viral culture or PCR. If initial swabs are negative patients should therefore be asked to re-attend immediately genital symptoms recur so that further swabs can be taken.

17.3 DIAGNOSIS OF GENITAL HERPES

17.3.1 Culture

Most laboratories are now able to perform herpes typing. This is of some prognostic significance regarding recurrence rate (see above) and can be helpful information when counseling patients.

The chances of obtaining a positive culture will depend very much on the stage of the lesion: ulcers shed more virus than crusting lesions. This needs to be explained to the patient who may not fully appreciate why they were diagnosed as having herpes at their initial consultation and then told a week or two later that their "herpes test" was negative. Some laboratories now perform PCR for diagnosing herpes infection. This is considered a much more sensitive method of diagnosis compared to viral culture.

17.3.2 Serology

Serological assays that distinguish between HSV type 1 and type 2 antibodies are now available but should be used selectively. Herpes serology is of no diagnostic value for primary herpes. Serology has a possible useful role in patients attending with recurrent genital ulceration and negative herpes culture. A negative result almost rules out herpes as a cause for the ulceration, although false negative results do occur, whereas a positive result for HSV type 2 antibody makes the diagnosis of genital herpes very likely.

Serology may also be helpful in couples where one partner has documented genital herpes and the other gives no history of infection. Positive HSV type 2 serology in the partner with no clinical history of herpes indicates previous infection and a degree of immunity, assuming that the infected partner has type 2 infection. This obviously reduces the anxiety associated with the possibility of herpes transmission during sexual intercourse. However, the converse must also be considered; a negative result may increase anxiety owing to concerns regarding the possibility of infecting the negative partner. Discussion with both partners is required and time given to consider the consequences.

Pregnant women with no history of genital herpes but with an infected partner may wish to avoid intercourse during the pregnancy if she proves HSV antibody negative (see section on "Pregnancy").

17.4 MANAGEMENT

17.4.1 Primary Genital Herpes

Women tend to fare rather worse than men. The genital sores are often exquisitely tender, urination may be intolerable, and patients usually feel generally very unwell with myalgia, headaches, fever, etc. The following are the recommended:

- Take a swab for herpes virus culture or PCR.
- Advise taking aspirin or paracetamol (or stronger preparation) as required.
- Bathe the genital area twice daily with warm salty water and dry with the hair dryer on cool setting.
- Some women find it easier to pass urine while sitting in a warm bath.
- Prescribe aciclovir tablets 200 mg five times a day for 5 days, famciclovir 250 mg tds for 5 days, or valaciclovir 500 mg bd for 5 days.
- There is no place for topical aciclovir cream in treating primary herpes.

Urinary retention secondary to sacral radiculopathy is uncommon and affects women and homosexual men more commonly than heterosexual men.

Approximately 10% of women suffer coincidental vaginal candidiasis. If there is generalized vulval erythema in addition to areas of ulceration or if symptoms persist after the ulcers have healed, consider treating for *Candida* with an oral agent such as fluconazole 150 mg stat dose or itraconazole 200 mg bd for 1 day. Most women are rather too sore to use pessaries or cream.

The diagnosis of herpes can be psychologically traumatic and a great deal of time is often required to provide adequate information about the disease. Some patients require further more intensive "counseling" to help them come to terms with the condition. Key issues which need to be addressed include the possibility of asymptomatic viral shedding, the effect this may have on current or future sexual relationships, and the use of condoms to provide some protection to sexual partners. The issue of herpes in pregnancy is discussed below.

17.4.2 Recurrent Herpes

Most patients cope extremely well with herpes. Attacks are usually infrequent and last only a few days and can be managed quite adequately by bathing the affected area with salty water and avoiding sexual contact while lesions are present.

A small number of patients suffer rather more painful and prolonged attacks and may benefit from a course of famciclovir (125 mg bd for 5 days), aciclovir tablets (200 mg five times a day for 3–5 days), valaciclovir 500 mg bd for 5 days or aciclovir cream (which must be used five times a day) taken or applied immediately when lesions appear. There has been some debate regarding the treatment of recurrent herpes with intermittent short courses of antiviral agents and concern raised about the possibility of generating resistant viral strains; however, this would appear to be more of an issue with immunosuppressed patients on long-term suppressive treatment. It is worth emphasizing that most patients with recurrent herpes do not require therapy.

For the small minority of patients who are plagued by very frequent and prolonged recurrences, it may be worth considering prophylactic therapy. This entails taking tablets on a daily basis for up to 1 year initially after which time the medication is stopped and the frequency of recurrences re-assessed. Current regimens include acyclovir 400 mg bd (a frequently used treatment), aciclovir 200 mg four times a day, famciclovir 250 mg bd, and valaciclovir 500 mg daily. Patients are usually reviewed at

3-monthly intervals. Viral shedding can occur whilst on suppressive treatment even in the absence of clinically obvious recurrences, a point worth mentioning to patients.

17.4.3 Pregnancy

Neonatal herpes carries a significant mortality and morbidity but is fortunately a rare condition in the UK. The baby is at greatest risk if the mother develops primary herpes during the last trimester, particularly toward the time of labor. Interestingly, recent studies have shown that most babies with neonatal herpes acquire their infection from mothers with asymptomatic primary herpes who are shedding virus during the birth.

There is minimal risk to the baby in women with recurrent disease. This is probably related to protective antibody passing across the placenta and to a much lower rate of viral shedding from the cervix in recurrent disease compared with primary infection. This is important to mention after diagnosing herpes as issues regarding future pregnancies are high on the list of worries. Women with a past history of genital herpes should be advised to present early in labor and undergo a careful examination for evidence of genital lesions. Although there is minimal risk to the baby, in view of the severity of neonatal herpes, most obstetricians would advise cesarean section rather than vaginal delivery if lesions are present. Daily aciclovir can be used in the last 4 weeks of pregnancy to reduce the risk of clinical recurrence and the need for cesarean section. Although aciclovir is not licensed for use in pregnancy, there is substantial evidence to support its safety.

The diagnosis and management of genital herpes can sometimes pose problems. Referral to GU medicine should therefore be considered even if it is just for discussion or to provide information.

17.5 OTHER CAUSES OF GENITAL ULCERATION

17.5.1 Candidiasis

Vulval candidiasis may occasionally be mistaken for genital herpes particularly when there is severe vulval soreness with disruption of the vulva epithelium. Conversely, recurrent herpes may produce only minor vulval discomfort and be dismissed by the patient as simply an attack of "thrush." For this reason it is important to explain to patients with a history of herpes that minor genital symptoms may be a recurrence of their herpes and that necessary care should be taken during sexual intercourse.

17.5.2 Syphilis

Syphilis is now making a reappearance in the UK and should be considered in all patients presenting with genital ulceration. The primary chancre of primary syphilis is usually painless, although secondary infection may produce some tenderness (Figure 17.5). Patients should be referred to GU medicine if there is the slightest doubt regarding the clinical diagnosis of genital ulceration. Dark-ground microscopy for treponemes can be performed on site and optimal specimens will be obtained for herpes culture. Remember that syphilis serology may be negative in primary syphilis, although *T. pallidum* IgM antibody should be requested if a chancre is considered a possible diagnosis. IgM should become detectable toward the second week of infection with IgG becoming positive at about 4 weeks. However, it is still prudent to advise patients with genital ulceration of unknown cause to have repeat syphilis serology performed at 3 months after presentation.

The chancre of primary syphilis may pass unnoticed and the patient presents with the generalized rash of secondary syphilis often associated with lymphadenopathy and fever. Syphilis should be considered in the differential diagnosis of patients presenting with a glandular fever like illness and while your history taking moves toward sexual contacts please also consider HIV seroconversion illness.

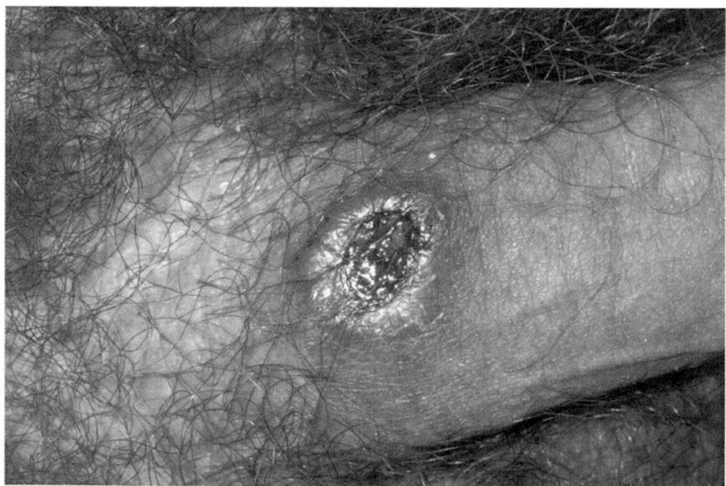

FIGURE 17.5. Chancre of primary syphilis affecting the penis

17.5.3 Fixed Drug Eruption

More severe cases may lead to ulceration (see Chapter 16, page 93).

17.5.4 Chancroid and Lymphogranuloma Venereum

These are common tropical STIs but rare in the UK, although cases of LGV proctitis amongst men who have sex with men have recently been reported in Western Europe, including the UK. Remember to ask about sexual contact with partners from abroad.

17.5.5 Aphthous Ulceration and Behçet's Disease

The genital ulcers in Behçet's disease are very tender and usually have a well-demarcated edge (Figure. 17.6). To make a diagnosis of Behçet's disease there should also be a history of oral ulceration together with eye, skin, or neurological complications.

In women, one more commonly sees simple aphthous ulceration affecting the mouth and labia, there being no other features to suggest Behçet's disease.

17.5.6 Trauma

Traumatic lesions are usually the result of forced sexual intercourse or rather too vigorous oral sex. The lesions often appear as abrasions rather than true ulcers; however, a swab for herpes

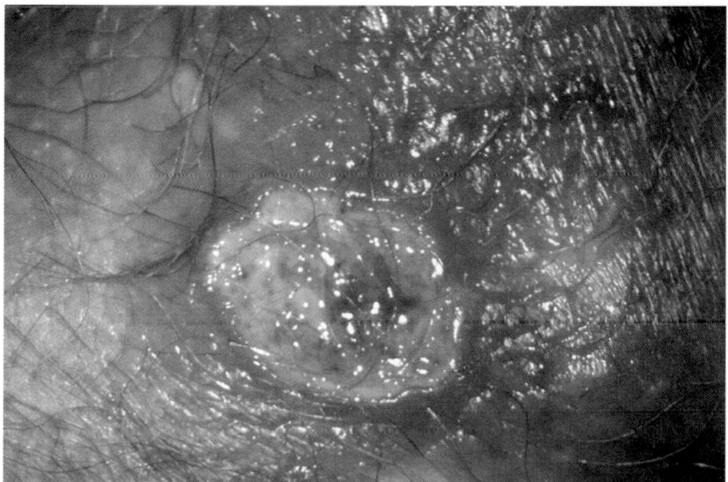

FIGURE 17.6. Genital ulcer of Behçet's syndrome (similar appearance with aphthous ulceration)

simplex virus culture should be performed as herpes may present in this fashion with the patient often under the misguided impression that the lesion was related to physical skin damage.

17.5.7 Ulcers of Lipschutz

In 1913, Lipschutz described cases of acute vulval ulceration associated with fever and lymphadenopathy. More recently, genital ulceration has been described as an uncommon complication of infectious mononucleosis and it is therefore possible that Lipschutz's original cases related to Epstein-Barr virus infection.

17.5.8 Bullous Skin Conditions

Pemphigus and cicatricial pemphigoid very occasionally present on the genitalia. The bullae may be short-lived leaving areas of eroded epithelium.

Any case of genital ulceration for which a definitive diagnosis cannot be made should ideally be referred to GU medicine for assessment and further investigation.

Chapter 18
Genital "Lumps"

18.1 GENITAL WARTS

The most frequently seen genital "lumps" in general practice are genital warts or condylomata acuminata ("pointed condylomata"). The term "venereal warts" is now outdated and should not be used. Genital warts are the second commonest STI in the UK and are caused by human papillomavirus (HPV), which is the commonest sexually transmitted viral infection in the UK. Studies using nucleic acid amplification tests (e.g. polymerase chain reaction) for detecting tiny amounts of HPV DNA suggest that many sexually active people carry low levels of HPV in the genital tract for variable periods of time but only a small number of infected individuals develop warts. The natural history and infectivity of this so-called "subclinical" HPV infection is unknown.

A prophylactic vaccine against HPV types 6,11,16 and 18 has recently been licensed in the USA and UK. This should provide protection against genital warts and many cases of cervical, vulval, anal and penile intraepithelial neoplasia and carcinoma.

18.1.1 Management of Genital Warts

Patients with genital warts should ideally be referred to GU medicine for assessment and initiation of treatment, irrespective of the age of the patient and the length of time the warts have been present. Genital warts are almost always sexually acquired (Figures 18.1–18.5), although lesions may have been present for many months or even years before the patient seeks a medical opinion. Very occasionally hand warts may be transferred to the genitalia and this should be considered if the lesions resemble planar warts rather than condylomata acuminata.

The incubation period between acquiring HPV infection and the appearance of warts may be many months or, very occasionally, even years, which can lead to some difficulty in determining exactly when and from whom the infection was caught.

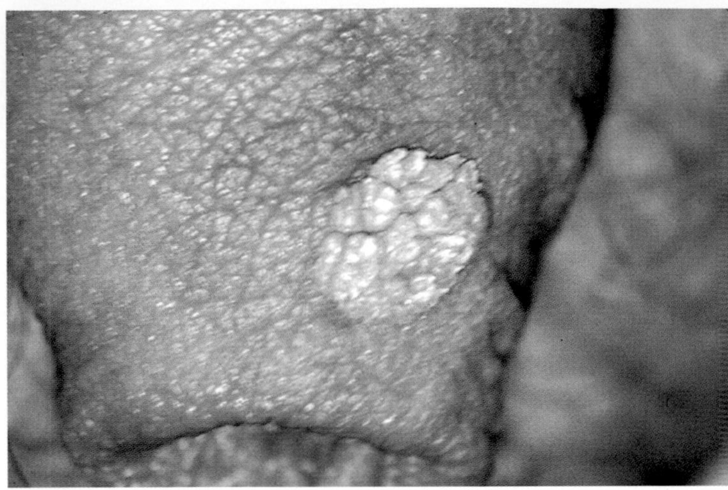

FIGURE 18.1. Penile wart

Anal warts (Figure 18.6) are commonly seen in both women and heterosexual men, either with or without genital lesions, and these may extend into the anal canal. Anal warts are not indicative

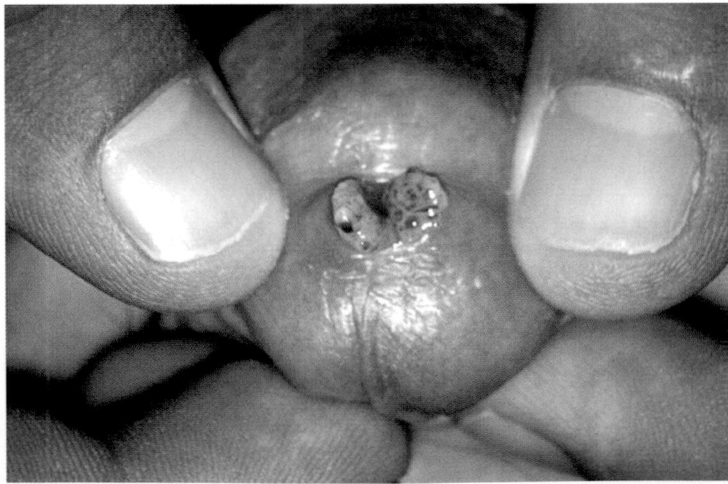

FIGURE 18.2. Intra-meatal wart

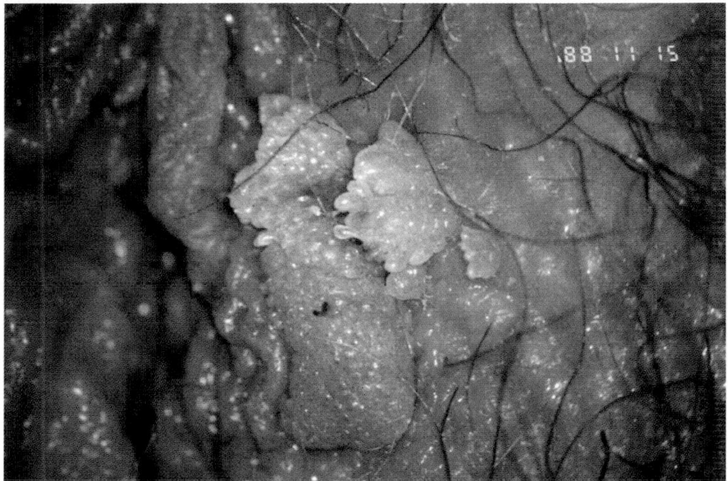

FIGURE 18.3. Vulval warts

of anal intercourse; the method by which HPV is transferred to the anus of a heterosexual male is currently unknown

HPV infection is sexually acquired and most patients should be checked for other STIs, in particular chlamydial infection.

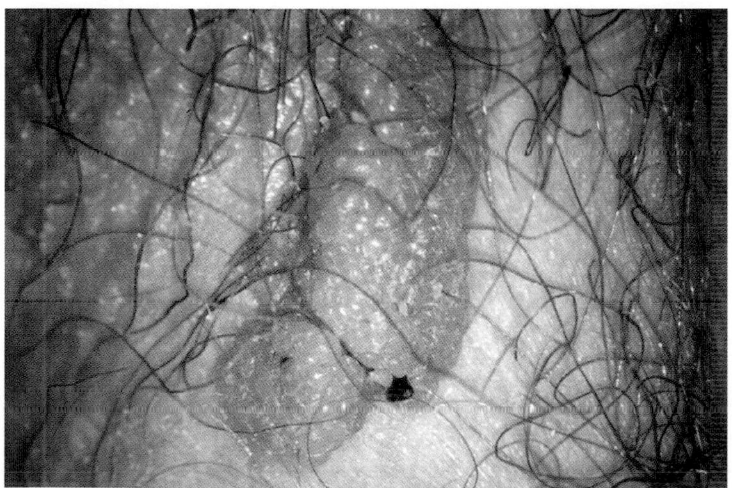

FIGURE 18.4. Keratinized vulval warts

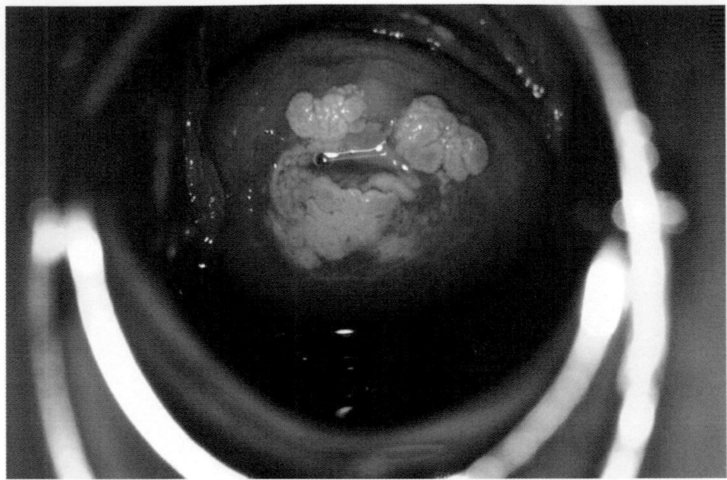

FIGURE 18.5. Cervical warts

Remember that STIs are frequently carried without symptoms. Sexual partners should be carefully assessed, which for female partners should include vaginal and cervical examination, ideally with a colposcope.

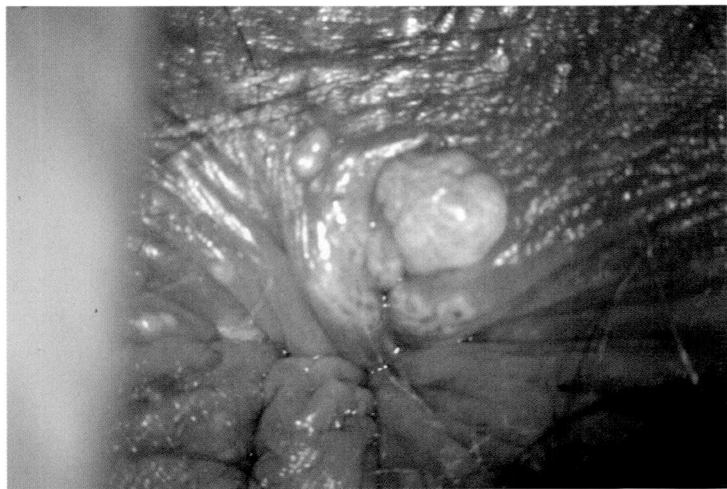

FIGURE 18.6. Anal warts

18.1.2 Treatment

(1) Cryotherapy is an extremely effective and generally well-tolerated treatment that does not require a local anesthetic. This is a useful first-line treatment.

(2) Podophyllin is a time-honored treatment that requires application by medical staff twice or thrice weekly. The patient should wash off the paint after 4–6 hours as prolonged application can lead to burning and ulceration. Fresh, moist warts may respond well to this form of treatment. Once keratin has started to appear on the wart surface success is less likely. Anecdotal evidence suggests that a combination of cryotherapy and topical podophyllin is more effective than either therapy alone. Podophyllin is now uncommonly used as sole therapy.

(3) Podophyllotoxin is a pure preparation of one of the active ingredients of podophyllin and has the advantage of self-application either as a lotion or as a cream. It is quite expensive compared with podophyllin but is highly effective in patients with fresh lesions and is ideal for those who find it difficult to adhere to regular clinic or surgery attendance. Some women find it difficult to apply, particularly if lesions are small, and treatment of anal warts usually requires some assistance.

(4) Imiquimod is also a self-applied cream that works by stimulating the cell-mediated immune response against HPV in the infected epithelium. As with podophyllotoxin, some patients experience soreness at the site of application. Response to treatment is sometimes a little slow, perhaps taking 8–12 weeks to act in some patients, but initial studies have suggested a lower recurrence rate than with other forms of treatment.

(5) Trichloracetic acid acts as a caustic agent and can be useful for burning off small warts. To be used with care!

(6) Diathermy, scissor excision and laser ablation require a local anesthetic; prior application of prilocaine plus lignocaine cream makes this more tolerable. Very useful for persistent warts and should be considered earlier rather than later in the course of treatment.

Since warts may resolve without treatment a "wait and see" approach may be considered. Unfortunately warts may enlarge and spread making treatment at a later date more difficult. In addition, most patients dislike the physical appearance of genital warts and usually opt for treatment.

The method of treatment used should be guided by lesion type, site, size, number, and patient needs. Single or small numbers of warts are effectively treated with cryotherapy or removal under local anesthetic whereas numerous lesions may be better approached with a self-applied treatment such as imiquimod or podophyllotoxin. More detailed advice is probably better sought from a specialist text (see Further Reading).

18.1.3 Other Management Issues and Frequently Asked Questions

18.1.3.1 Recurrences

Genital warts have a tendency to recur, in some cases with alarming frequency. Such patients may require psychological support.

18.1.4 HPV Infection and Anogenital Cancer

There is now a good deal of evidence linking HPV infection with cervical, vulval, penile, and anal squamous cell carcinoma. Most studies have focused on cervical neoplasia and dysplasia (or CIN) and have shown certain HPV types to have a greater potential to induce dysplastic and neoplastic change. The commonest so-called "high risk" types are HPV-16 and 18. HPV-6 and 11 are found in genital warts and are considered "low-risk" HPV types. As mentioned earlier, many sexually active people harbor low levels of HPV in the genital tract, including the high-risk types 16 or 18. In most individuals this infection probably eventually clears, in others it may persist indefinitely but pose no problem. In a small number of individuals, HPV infection may induce cellular dysplastic change. Dysplasia may revert to normal over time or, again in a small number of individuals, progress to cancer. The chances of an individual infected with a "high-risk" HPV type developing a cervical cancer depends on several factors. These include the quantity of virus present, the genetically determined immunological host response to the virus, which will have some control over viral persistence, and other cofactors such as smoking, herpes simplex virus co-infection and possibly the presence of other genital infections (e.g. *Chlamydia*). Current UK guidelines do not advise more frequent cervical cytology in women with a history of genital warts or genital wart contact.

18.1.5 Condom Use

Most clinicians advise the use of condoms while warts are present and most patients feel comfortable with this. Although HPV remains in the epithelium after warts have cleared, the degree of infectivity of subclinically carried virus is currently unknown as is the protective effect of condoms for subclinical infection. It is therefore very difficult to accurately advise for how long condoms should be used after apparently successful treatment. There would appear to be less need to use condoms in long-term relationships as the exposed partner is likely to have already been infected with the virus.

18.1.6 Oral Sex

As warts can occasionally be passed to the mouth through oro-genital contact, it is usually recommended that couples refrain from oral sex whilst warts are present. However, depending upon the site and extent of lesions, with sufficient care it may be possible to avoid direct wart contact.

18.2 OTHER CAUSES OF GENITAL "LUMPS"

18.2.1 Hirsuties Papillaris Penis Or Pearly Penile Papules

"Hirsuties papillaris penis" or "penile pearly pink papules" is one of the commonest conditions to be mistaken for genital warts in men. The lesions appear as rows of small pink or white filiform papillae on the corona of the glans penis and by the frenulum (Figure 18.7). They first appear at puberty and are found to varying degrees in up to 40% of men. They are harmless but a frequent cause of anxiety; if you are unsure, ask GU medicine to

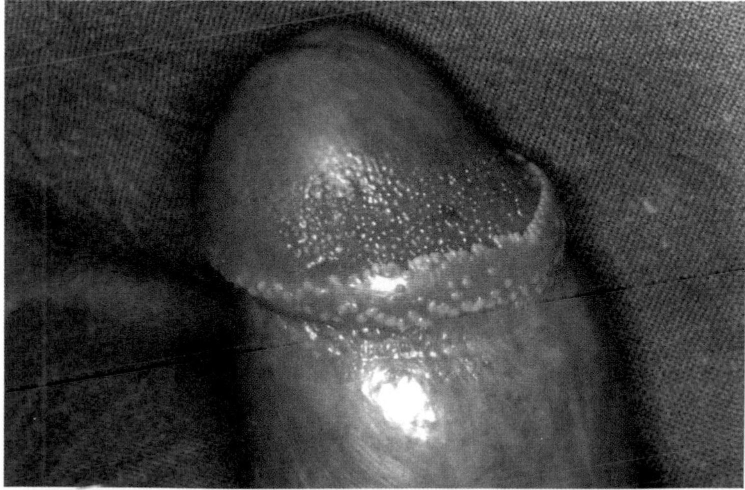

FIGURE 18.7. Hirsuties papillaris penis (penile papules)

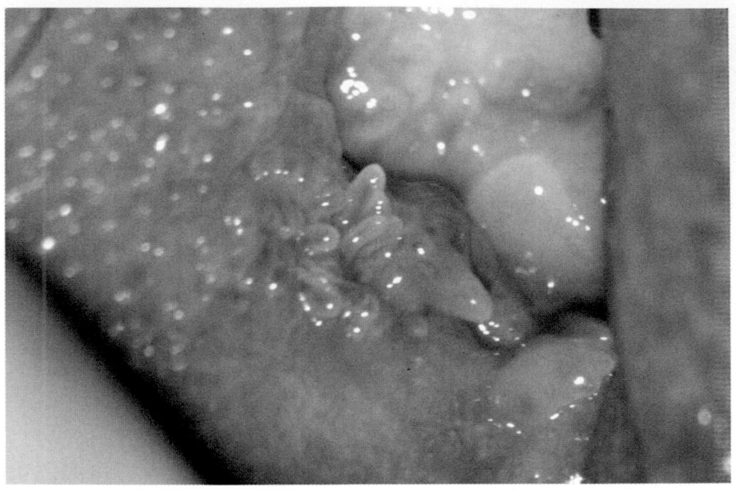

FIGURE 18.8. Vulval micropapillae

assess. Tiny papules by the frenulum can be difficult to distinguish from warts and may require examination with the aid of a magnifying glass or colposcope.

Penile papules can be removed by cryotherapy or laser ablation if causing sufficient cosmetic anxiety but reassurance is usually sufficient.

18.2.2 Vulval Micropapillae

Many women have small finger-like projections on the inner surface of the labia minora and around the introitus. These are benign micropapillae (Figure 18.8) and may be seen in conjunction with warts, which often makes clinical assessment difficult. Micropapillae are not related to HPV infection and therefore do not warrant treatment. Examination with some form of magnification, such as the colposcope, is often required to differentiate these lesions from genital warts.

18.2.3 Fordyce Spots

"Fordyce spots" (Figures 18. 9 and 18.10) are commonly seen in both men and women. They are a normal variant, thought to be ectopic sebaceous glands, which appear as tiny cream-colored spots just under the skin surface.

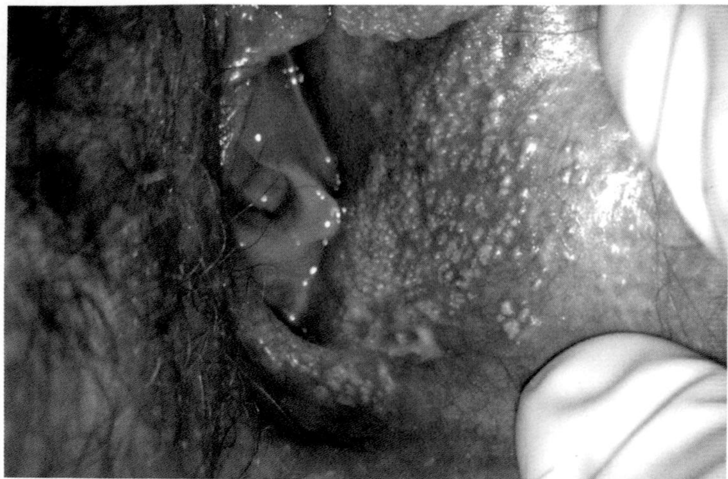

FIGURE 18.9. Vulval Fordyce spots

18.2.4 Pilo-Sebaceous Glands

These are commonly found along the penile shaft but in some men they can be particularly numerous and prominent, giving rise to concern. The patient should be reassured that these are normal skin glands and do not require treatment (Figure 18.11).

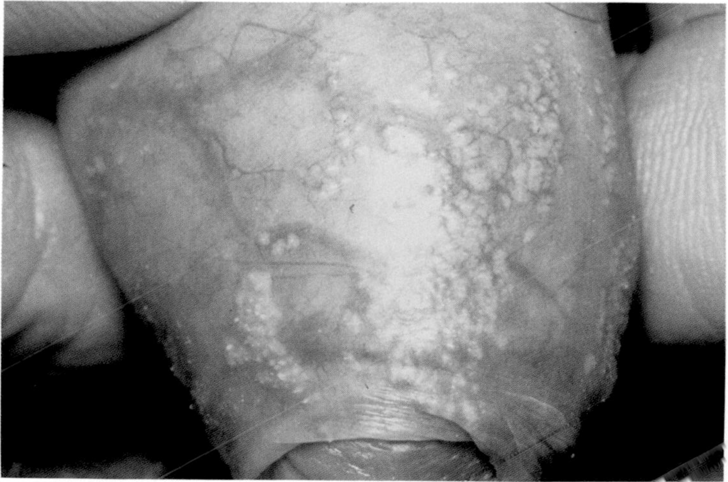

FIGURE 18.10. Penile Fordyce spots

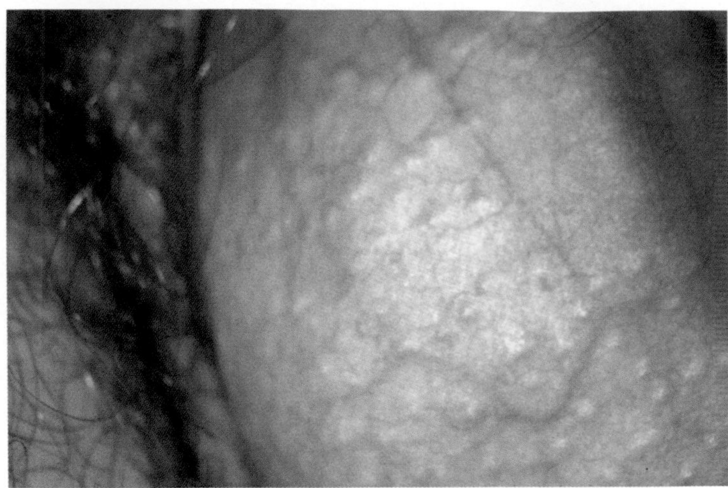

FIGURE 18.11. Prominent pilo-sebaceous glands on the penile shaft

18.2.5 Seborrhoeic Keratoses

These more commonly appear with increasing age and may resemble warts. Removal by curettage, scissor or shave excision under local anaesthetic for histological examination is recommeded if there is diagnostic uncertainty. Cryotherapy is an alternative effective method of treatment (Figure 18.12).

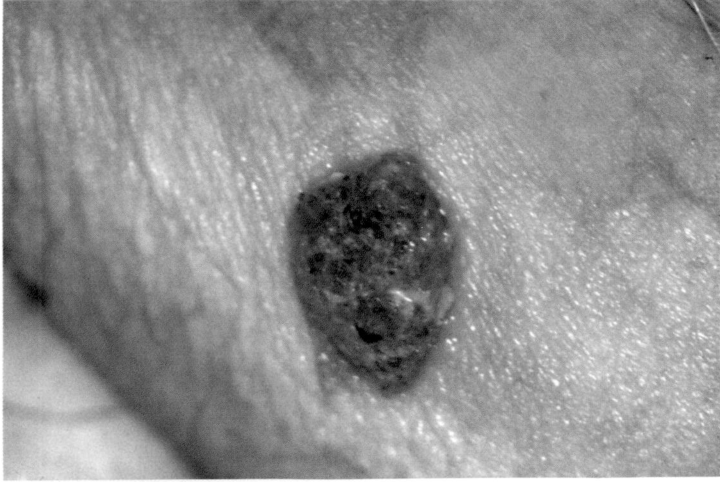

FIGURE 18.12. Seborrhoeic keratoses

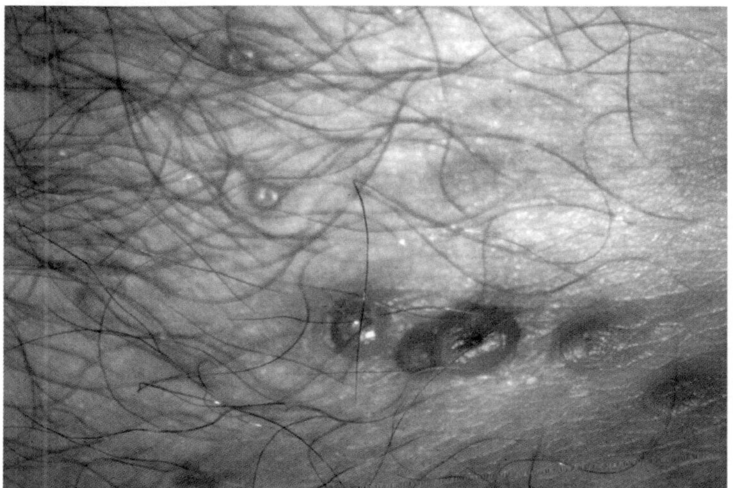

FIGURE 18.13. Molluscum contagiosum

18.2.6 Molluscum Contagiosum

Lesions are classically smooth and rounded with a central punctum although polypoid forms are occasionally seen (Figure 18.13). Treatment is with cryotherapy. Applying phenol with a sharpened orange stick tends to be less well tolerated. Recent reports have also shown promising results using imiquimod, podophyllotoxin and cidofovir.

18.2.7 Sebaceous Cysts

These present as round, creamy yellow, smooth swellings. Scrotal cysts may reach a centimeter in diameter and are often multiple (Figure 18.14).

18.2.8 Lichen Planus

Papular lesions of lichen planus may be mistaken for flat or papular warts. Diagnosis is aided by the violaceous color and the presence of fine white linear striae (Wickham's striae) and by the presence of the condition elsewhere on the body (see also page 90 figure 18.5).

18.2.9 Linchen Nitidus

An uncommon condition presenting as very tiny pink or brown, dome-shaped, shiny papules. They may be found in conjunction with lichen planus.

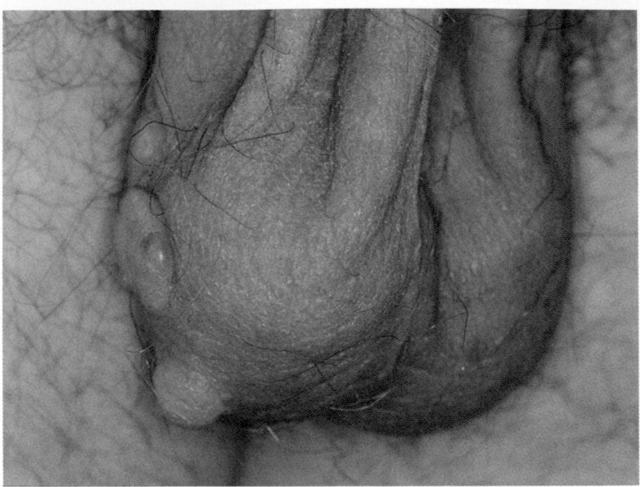

FIGURE 18.14. Scrotal sebaceous cysts

18.4.1 Psoriasis

Plaques of psoriasis may occasionally be misdiagnosed as flat warts. Genital lesions often lack the characteristic silvery scale leaving a red, slightly shiny surface (see also page 91 figure 16.6).

18.4.2 Condylomata Lata

A feature of secondary syphilis that presents as pink or grey, moist, slightly elevated lesions (Figure 18.15). There are often other signs of syphilis (e.g. generalized rash, oral lesions, lymphadenopathy) and syphilis serology (*T. pallidum* antibody; VDRL (Venereal Diseases Research Laboratories) and TPHA (*T. pallidum* hemagglutination assay)) will be positive at this stage of the disease.

18.4.3 PIN and Squamous Cell Carcinoma

Penile intraepithelial neoplasia presents as a flat or papular, erythematous or whitish, warty looking lesion (Figure 18.16 and page 92 figure 16.9). The application of acetic acid (gauze swab soaked in 5% acetic acid and held against the lesion for 3–5 minutes) highlights the lesions, although examination with a colposcope may be needed to reveal the characteristic features of punctation. Biopsy is required to confirm the clinical diagnosis. PIN is a pre-malignant condition. Cancerous lesions usually feel hard or gritty, often bleed on contact, and may be ulcerated. Genital warts rarely undergo malignant change but any suspicious lesion requires biopsy.

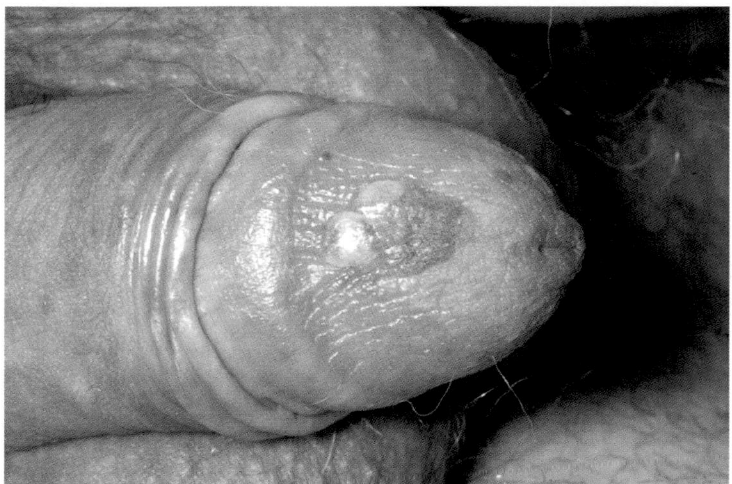

FIGURE 18.15. Condylomata lata of secondary syphilis

18.4.4 Lymphocele

A common condition presenting as a smooth, firm, worm-like cord in or below the coronal sulcus just below the glans penis. There may be a history of recent strenuous sexual activity. There is no specific treatment and the condition resolves with time (Figure 18.17).

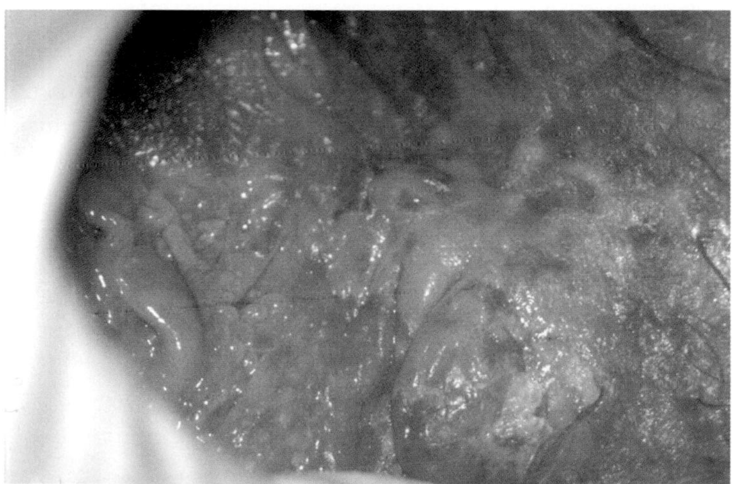

FIGURE 18.16. Penile intraepithelial neoplasia (PIN)

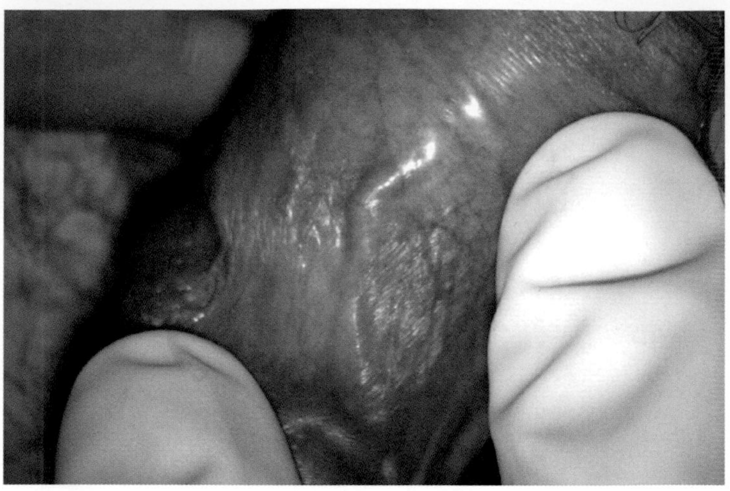

FIGURE 18.17. Penile lymphocoele

18.4.5 Peyronie's Disease

A condition of unknown cause characterized by the development of fibrous plaques *within* the penis. Some patients give a history of penile trauma which is thought to allow bleeding into the tunica albuginea. This initiates an inflammatory reaction that leads to fibrin deposition and scar formation. The first sign noted by the patient is often a painless lump, sometimes associated with discomfort on erection. As the condition progresses, the penis may bend to one side on erection, occasionally making intercourse impossible. Some patients notice the penile bending before a lump is detected. There is usually spontaneous improvement with time (often months or years) and reassurance may be all that is required. Potassium para-aminobenzoate (POTABA) and vitamin E combined with colchicine and intralesional verapamil or triamcinolone injection have been tried, with variable success in the early acute phase of the disease. Surgery is best reserved for those patients with a penile deformity that interferes with intercourse.

Chapter 19
Genital Irritation

The patient presenting with genital irritation should be asked the following:

- *Exactly where is the irritation* – penis, scrotum, toward the entrance of the vagina, on the labia majora, above the genitalia in the public area?
- Is there anything to see, such as a rash, warts, or public lice?
- Is there irritation elsewhere on the body?

The following are the commonest causes of genital irritation:

- *Dermatoses* – dermatitis, lichen simplex, lichen planus, lichen sclerosus, etc.
- *Infection* – candidiasis, early genital herpes (preulcerative stage), HPV infection (warts or VIN), trichomoniasis, pubic lice.

These conditions are mostly covered in other sections (see Chapters 8 and 16). This chapter will focus on the two common parasitic infections: pubic lice and scabies.

19.1 PUBIC LICE ("CRABS" OR PEDICULOSIS)

The pubic louse (*Phthirus pubis*) may spread to any hairy part of the body with the exception of the scalp and eyebrows. Very occasionally the eyelashes may be involved. Transmission is by body contact although toilet seats and shared clothing have been implicated in a small number of cases. Pubic lice are very slow movers and live for only a day away from the host.

19.1.1 Symptoms

Irritation is the commonest presenting symptom and the severity will depend on the level of hypersensitivity to mite antigen. In a previously unexposed individual, symptoms may take up to 5 days to occur. Excessive scratching can sometimes lead to excoriation and secondary infection. A large infestation resulting in multiple bites over a short period of time may cause mild fever and general malaise.

19.1.2 Signs

A careful search for eggs (nits) and lice may be required in milder infections. To the uninitiated, lice resemble "freckles" or small brown "scabs" (Figure 19.1). Pubic lice move on average a maximum of only 10 cm a day so it is unusual to see any activity during a 5-minute consultation.

19.1.3 Management

Clothing should be laundered in hot water or by dry cleaning.

The most widely used pediculosides are 0.5% malathion lotion, 1% permethrin cream, 0.2% phenothrin, and 0.5% or 1% carbaryl. Preparations are usually rubbed into the hairs and washed off 12 hours later. Although a second treatment is recommended after 1 week to kill any lice emerging from surviving eggs, the presence of eggs does not signify treatment failure. The possibility of itching persisting after successful treatment should be mentioned to the patient. If this proves a problem, consider using topical hydrocortisone or an oral antihistamine, such as one of the sedative preparations, at night.

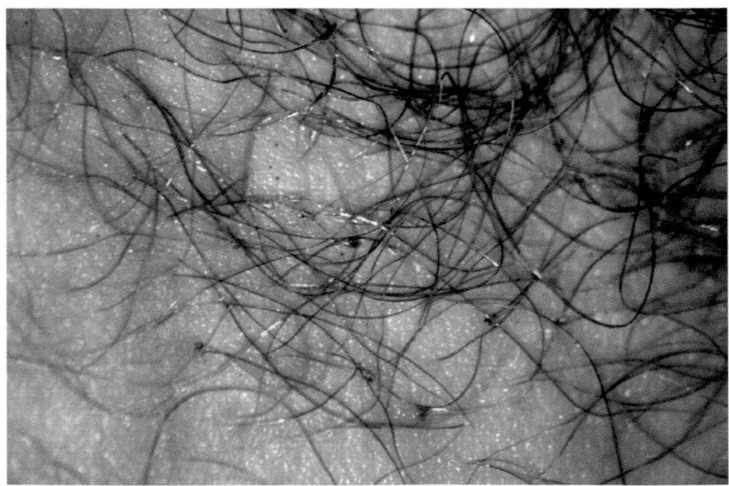

FIGURE 19.1. Pubic lice and nits (seen as tiny brown 'marks') – may be difficult to visualise in mild infections

Shaving the hair is unnecessary and may aggravate the irritation. Sexual contacts should be assessed and treated as appropriate. An infestation affecting the eyelashes may be effectively treated with permethrin or by applying Vaseline gently to the lashes.

19.2 SCABIES

The scabies mite (*Sarcoptes scabei*) is much smaller than the pubic louse and is only just visible to the naked eye. Transmission is by close personal contact and occasionally by wearing infected clothes. Although scabies is seen in school-age children, transmission within schools is uncommon. Outbreaks occasionally occur in nursing homes, hospitals, and other institutions. The incubation period for a first attack is up to 8 weeks with subsequent attacks producing symptoms within a few days because of previous sensitization.

19.2.1 Symptoms

Irritation tends to be generalized, sparing the head, and is worse at night.

DRI LIBRARY SERVICE WITHDRAWN FROM STOCK

19.2.2 Signs

Genital lesions are generally found only in men and appear as nodules on the penile shaft and scrotum. There is usually evidence of scabies elsewhere, particularly favored sites being the finger webs and sides of the fingers, flexor surfaces of the wrists, extensor surfaces of the elbows, anterior axillary folds, umbilicus, nipples, and buttock creases.

Classical lesions include the following:

- Short, wavy, dirty appearing burrows
- Small, erythematous, eczematous papules
- Small nodules (penis, scrotum) (Figure 19.2).

The scalp, face, and neck are spared in adults. Scratch marks are frequently seen and secondary eczematization and infection may mask the other features and make diagnosis rather more difficult.

19.2.3 Diagnosis

Scabies is often diagnosed purely on clinical grounds: intense irritation, especially at night, characteristic lesions, and similar complaints in household members or sexual partners. Where possible, however, an attempt should be made to confirm the diagnosis which involves identifying the mite, eggs, or larvae

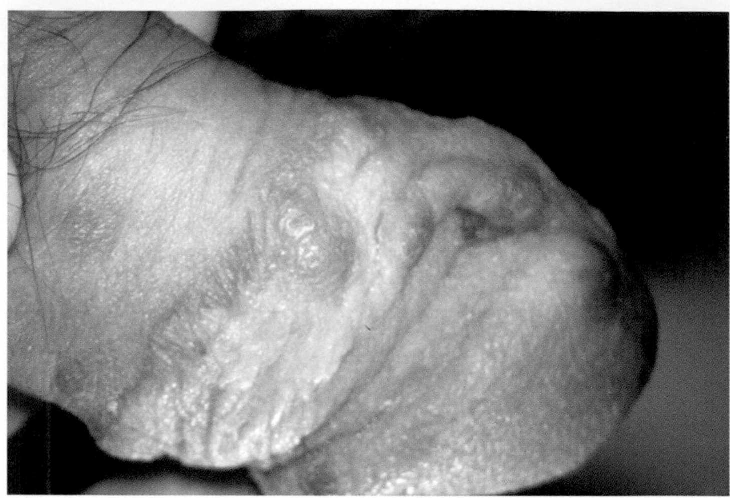

FIGURE 19.2. Scabetic nodules

under the microscope. First place a drop or two of Indian ink on to a suspected burrow and remove any excess with an alcohol wipe. This helps to "highlight" the burrow which should then be scraped gently with a scalpel blade and the material obtained transferred to a microscope slide. Apply a cover slip and examine with a microscope using low-power magnification.

19.2.4 Management

(1) All household members and sexual partners should be treated: they may remain asymptomatic for up to 8 weeks and during that time spread the disease unknowingly.
(2) All patients should be warned to expect continued irritation for as long as 3 months after successful treatment.
(3) Warn patients against overtreatment that can cause an irritant dermatitis.
(4) Lotions are easier to apply than creams.
(5) The lotion should be applied to all of the skin from the neck downward with particular attention to palms, soles, interdigital spaces, and genitals. This is most easily performed with a 3–5 cm paint brush and help is usually required to reach the more distant areas.
(6) Bathing before the lotion is applied is unnecessary and may increase systemic absorption of the scabicide.

(7) Antihistamines and crotamiton cream may help to relieve the irritation.
(8) Re-infection from bedlinen and clothing is no longer considered a risk.

The treatments available include 0.5% malathion lotion and 5% permethrin cream. These should be washed off after 24 hours.

Chapter 20

Human Immunodeficiency Virus (HIV) Infection

In the UK, GU medicine physicians provide much of the outpatient care, and in some hospitals also the in-patient care, for patients with HIV infection. The diagnosis still carries a certain stigma and may bring to the forefront emotions regarding past sexual relationships, sexuality, or drug abuse. In the 1980s, AIDS received a tremendous amount of hype by "medical" journalists and social commentators but with advances in our knowledge of the disease and developments in treatment, HIV infection should now probably be better viewed as a chronic illness. Primary care practitioners are playing more of a role in managing patients with HIV infection, particularly during the pre-treatment years. However, once the disease progresses and highly active antiretroviral treatment (HAART) is considered necessary, specialist input should be sought. Inappropriate drug combinations can seriously limit future treatment strategies through the development of drug resistance, and choosing the right therapy for an individual patient is not always a straightforward matter. This chapter deals with just a few of the important issues regarding HIV antibody testing and patient management.

20.1 HIV ANTIBODY TESTING

(1) Many people request an HIV antibody test for "peace of mind". They may be entering a new sexual relationship and wish to clear up a nagging doubt about a previous partner. It is important to try and assess the degree of risk: Has there been previous sexual contact with bisexual or homosexual men, injecting drug users, or persons from "highrisk" areas of the world? Of course one can never be certain about the behavioral history of their previous partners and so direct questioning only provides a rough guide to the true risk. Although an unexpected positive result occasionally turns up, more commonly there is a clue from the history. Remember

that injecting users who deny ever sharing needles and syringes ("works") may have been exposed to HIV from their sexual partners who do share needles.

(2) Following infection with HIV, there is a delay of between 3 and 6 months before antibodies become detectable on serology. This "window period" needs to be explained to the patient and testing possibly delayed until sufficient time has elapsed after potential exposure. For this reason, testing is usually performed at 3 months after exposure. This may be repeated at 6 months in individuals who report known HIV exposure or have received post exposure prophylaxis with anti-retrovirals. Seroconversion after 6 months has been reported but is considered a rare event. Improved antibody detection tests and PCR have lessened the interval to detect infection and should be discussed with your local laboratory in cases where there is confirmed exposure to HIV.

(3) The "HIV antibody test" has become much more of a routine investigation and should be considered as such; however, a positive result does carry implications. It is therefore wise that the test is discussed, covering the points mentioned above, and the reason for testing explained in cases where HIV is on the list of differential diagnoses in a symptomatic patient.

(4) Although needle-stick injuries are more common in the hospital setting, occasionally the GP will be consulted following an injury in the community or in the surgery. The risk of acquiring HIV from a needle-stick injury from an infected-patient not taking anti-retrovivals is approximately 3%. The risk of transmission following an injury from a needle of "unknown origin" is obviously less. The risk of acquiring hepatitis B following a needle-stick injury from an "e antigen" positive patient is 30% and the risk of hepatitis C infection from a needle-stick injury is approximately 3%. If the injury were sustained by a doctor or nurse from a patient in the surgery, direct questioning will help to determine the risk of infection, although bear in mind that questions regarding sexuality and drug use may not always be answered honestly and that some infected patients give no history of "risk contact" If there is concern, ask the patient whether they would consent to being tested for HIV, hepatitis B and, if intravenous drug misuse is suspected, hepatitis C infection. If consent is denied and there is a definite risk of infection, consider a booster dose of hepatitis B vaccine, assuming that the healthcare worker has been previously vaccinated and that antibody levels are unknown. HIV serology should be performed at 3 and 6 months and condoms used during this time.

Specific hepatitis B immunoglobulin (HBIG) in addition to hepatitis B vaccination should be considered for patients sustaining a needle-stick injury in the community. A careful evaluation is required in each case to determine the true risk and whether prophylaxis is needed. If in doubt, err on the side of caution. HBIG should be given preferably within 48 hours and not later than a week after exposure at a dose of 200 IU for children of 0-4 years, 300 IU for children of 5–9 years and 500 IU for adults and children over 10 years. HIV serology should be performed at 3 and 6 months (see page 128 regarding earlier detection). Discussion with your local Public Health Laboratory is advisable; they may already have guidelines for the management of needle-stick injuries in general practice.

(5) Post exposure prophylaxis (PEP) should be strongly considered if there is needle-stick injury involving HIV infected blood, as does occasionally happen in the clinical setting. Three drugs are administered as soon as possible after the injury (ideally within 24 hours) although some practitioners will consider PEP up to two weeks after exposure. PEP is usually continued for 4–6 weeks. Prophylaxis post sexual exposure is also now considered worthwhile, the common scenario being a condom split or slippage in a discordant relationship (i.e. one partner HIV positive and the other negative). The decision to start PEP is not always straightforward (e.g. has the HIV infected person drug resistant virus, is the viral load undetectable, as is usually the case when on treatment, or is it very high, etc.) and specialist advice should be sought.

(6) Insurance companies used to ask new clients to state whether they had previously had an HIV antibody test or considered themselves at potential risk of acquiring HIV, whereas now they should only inquire whether there has been a previous positive test for HIV. Having previously been tested negative for HIV should no longer cause difficulties when applying for life insurance.

(7) Some "HIV-workers" have suggested that HIV pretest counseling should be performed only by experienced counselors within departments of GU medicine or by specialized testing centers. This is a rather extreme and outdated view. There is no reason why HIV antibody testing should not be performed in general practice; however, there are a few points worth considering. First, for reasons of confidentiality, many patients prefer not to have a record of HIV antibody testing in their general practice notes. If the result proves positive then of course it is important that the general practitioner is aware of the diagnosis. Secondly, patients with possible risk

factors for infection may be better assessed and tested in the GU medicine setting where full support and information can be provided if the result is positive. Thirdly, if an individual is concerned about possible sexual exposure to HIV then it is wise to check for other sexually transmitted infections, such as *Chlamydia*, which are far more common than HIV.

(8) Many GU medicine clinics now run "fast service" HIV antibody testing that provides results within 24 hours. This is ideal for the anxious patient who is deterred from testing because of a several day wait for results.

20.2 CLINICAL FEATURES AND MANAGEMENT

20.2.1 Seroconversion Illness

Over 50% of patients report a "flulike" or "glandular-fever like" illness at the time of seroconversion (i.e. about 2-6 months after infection).

20.2.2 Persistent Generalized Lymphadenopathy

After a variable period of time a number of patients develop cervical and axillary lymphadenopathy. This is usually painless and the glands affected are usually >1 cm in diameter. Lymphadenopathy is of no prognostic significance.

20.2.3 Constitutional Symptoms

Most patients with HIV remain asymptomatic for a number of years. During this time the virus is replicating in the lymphoid tissue and other body sites and although the CD4 or T-helper lymphocytes are being destroyed, the immune system is sufficiently robust to maintain normal lymphocyte levels. After a period of usually some years, the immune system shows signs of deterioration and the CD4 lymphocyte count falls. This is sometimes associated with the development of constitutional symptoms such as loss of weight, night sweats, diarrhea, and profound lethargy. It is important to remember, however, that many patients with low CD4 cell counts are asymptomatic. Symptoms of constitutional HIV disease improve with antiretroviral medication.

20.2.4 Acquired Immunodeficiency Syndrome (AIDS)

This is an emotive and not particularly helpful term clinically. A diagnosis of AIDS indicates marked immunosuppression and a number of clinical conditions ('indicator disease') will place the patient in the diagnostic category of AIDS. In addition, all persons with a CD4 lymphocyte count $<200 \times 10^6/l$ irrespective

Table 20.1. AIDS Defining Conditions (1993 classification).

Bacterial pneumonia (recurrent)
Candidiasis (esophageal, tracheal or bronchial; not oral)
CD4 lymphocyte count <200/mm^3
Cervical cancer (carcinoma in situ is not included)
Coccidiomycosis (disseminated or extrapulmonary)
Cryptococcal meningitis and other extrapulmonary disease
Cryptosporidiosis with diarrhea persisting for >1 month
Cytomegalovirus disease (other than liver, spleen, or lymph nodes)
Herpes simplex infection: ulceration persisting for longer than one month, bronchitis, pneumonitis, esophagitis
HIV encephalopathy
HIV wasting syndrome
Histoplasmosis (disseminated or extrapulmonary)
Isosporiasis with diarrhea persisting for >1 month
Kaposi's sarcoma
Lymphoma of the brain
Non-Hodgkin's lymphoma
Mycobacterium avium complex disease
Mycobacterium tuberculosis: any site (pulmonary or extrapulmonary)
Mycobacterium of other species: disseminated or extrapulmonary
Pneumocystis carinii pneumonia (PCP)
Progressive multifocal leucoencephalopathy
Salmonella septicemia (recurrent)
Toxoplasmosis of the brain

of the presence or absence of an 'indicatior disease' are now classified as having AIDS. However, it is important to reassure the patient that HARRT will often lead to dramatic clinical improvement, although this obviously will depend upon the severity of the AIDS defining illness. A small subgroup of patients with HIV remains clinically well for many years, which is probably the result of infection with a less virulent strain of virus. AIDS defining conditions are listed in Table 20.1.

20.2.5 Important Management Points

(1) Clinical review every 3–6 months is advisable. When patients are well the fewer visits to the clinic the better as it often serves as an unhappy reminder of their diagnosis. A great deal of psychological support, however, may be required for the patient and, in many cases, sexual partners and the immediate family. This is particularly important at the time of diagnosis and during the early months after diagnosis.

(2) Issues which should be addressed and discussed include the following:

(a) *Need to notify sexual or "works-sharing" partners.* This is an important issue that requires careful discussion. Partner notification is one of the many tasks performed by the GU medicine clinic health adviser and should be considered when a patient is reluctant to contact a previous partner directly. Most patients, however, fully appreciate the need to inform previous contacts and take on this responsibility.

(b) *How to avoid passing on the infection (i.e. what sexual practices are safe or unsafe; safe-injecting practices).* Condoms provide an adequate barrier to HIV; however, problems arise when they are not used consistently or when they split or slip off the penis. Extra strong condoms are available for anal intercourse, although these may occasionally tear, and remember to advise the use of water-based rather than oil-based lubricants (see Chapter 12).

There is a small but definite risk of transmitting HIV through oral sex; advise the use of a dental dam (a thin latex square) or flavored condoms.

Practices which may draw blood, such as biting or scratching, should be avoided.

Kissing, mutual masturbation, and body-rubbing are considered safe. Injecting drug users should avoid sharing contaminated needles, spoons, and syringes ("works") and many pharmacists and drug agencies now run needle-exchange schemes. Boiling used syringes and needles is a less safe alternative. Flushing "works" with bleach reduces levels of active virus but is unreliable and should only be considered when there is no reasonable alternative. Full-strength household bleach is required with a minimum contact time of 30 seconds.

(c) *Who should be informed or needs to know the diagnosis.* Advise the patient to think carefully before telling others of the diagnosis. Employers and work colleagues rarely need to be informed.

(d) *Healthy lifestyle.* This involves getting enough rest, taking exercise as tolerated, reducing and eventually stopping smoking, eating a "healthy" diet, and reducing unnecessary stress. Some patients benefit from complementary medical care such as reflexology, aromatherapy, facial massage, and relaxation and visualization techniques.

(e) *Pregnancy and the risk to the infant.* Most mother to baby transmission occurs late in pregnancy or during delivery. Without treatment, transmission rates vary from 15 to 20% in Europe and are higher, in the region of 30%, in Africa. With treatment the risk of transmission may be reduced to less than 1%. An increased risk of transmission to the baby is associated with a high maternal viral load, low CD4 lymphocyte count, premature rupture of membranes, and vaginal delivery with a detectable viral load. It is current practice to advise taking antiretroviral treatment during the later stages of pregnancy, either as a single agent (zidovudine) or as a triple drug regimen. Vaginal delivery may be considered if the viral load is below $50/mm^3$, otherwise an elective cesarean section is recommended at 38 weeks. The baby will also usually be prescribed zidovudine syrup for 4–6 weeks. Breast-feeding carries an additional risk of transmission and should be advised against where there are safe alternatives. Breast-feeding, however, is still recommended in the developing world where the protection against infectious disease outweighs the risk of HIV transmission.

(f) *What support is available.* Support will be available at both local and national level. Information about local support groups is best obtained from your local GU medicine clinic.

(g) *Immunization.* BCG and yellow fever vaccination should be avoided. Live attenuated vaccines for measles, mumps, rubella, and polio may be given, although it should be noted that polio virus may be excreted for longer periods than in uninfected persons.

Although pneumococcal vaccination has been recommended for HIV-positive patients, clinical efficacy has not been proven.

Further information on vaccination in the UK may be obtained from the HMSO publication *Immunisation against Infectious Disease.*

(h) *Clinical follow-up.* The importance of clinical follow-up should be stressed and an emphasis placed on the role of drugs to prevent complications, slow disease progression, and restore immune function.

(3) Baseline investigations performed routinely after diagnosis include the following:

- Confirmatory HIV antibody test
- HIV mRNA level (also known as the "viral load")

- Viral genotyping (also known as "drug resistance testing" - infection with a partially resistant virus is now common and will influence which drugs to use when starting HAART)
- Full blood count
- T lymphocyte subsets (CD4 and CD8)
- Liver function tests
- Fasting lipids (a number of antiretroviral drugs raise lipid levels)
- Hepatitis B and C serology
- Syphilis serology
- Toxoplasma serology
- Cytomegalovirus serology
- Chest radiograph
- Weight

(4) The CD4 lymphocyte count, CD4 percentage and "viral load" should be measured on a regular basis as this provides some guide to immune status. Every six months is usually sufficient in the early stage of infection if the CD4 count is high. More frequent monitoring is required when the CD4 count or percentage starts to decline as the decision to start HAART will be determined by the rate of decline or the level reached. The risk of developing *Pneumocystis carinii* pneumonia (PCP) increases once the CD4 count falls below 200/mm^3 and HAART should be started before this time. Most clinicians consider treatment as the count drops below 350/mm^3 and moves toward, but before it reaches, 200/mm^3. HAART would also be considered in symptomatic patients irrespective of the CD4 count. Prophylaxis against PCP is recommended for patients with CD4 counts below 200/mm^3 (e.g. cotrimoxazole 960 mg orally three times a week).

(5) HAART involves the use of a combination of drugs that act at various stages of the HIV replicative cycle. Three drugs are usually used initially, occasionally four, and a number of formulations combine drugs in a single tablet or capsule, to aid compliance. There are roughly three groups of commonly used drugs: nucleoside analogue reverse transcriptase inhibitors (e.g. zidovudine, didanosine, lamivudine, emtricitabine, tenofovir), non-nucleoside analogue reverse transcriptase inhibitors (e.g. efavirenz, nevirapine), and protease inhibitors (e.g. saquinavir, ritonavir, loprenavir/ritonavir, atazanavir/ritonovir, nelfinavir). As mentioned above, choosing the right combination for the individual patient is not always straightforward. Potential interactions with other medications, HIV drug resistance, patient lifestyle, other current medical problems (e.g. depression, anemia, hyperlipidemia) all need to be considered.

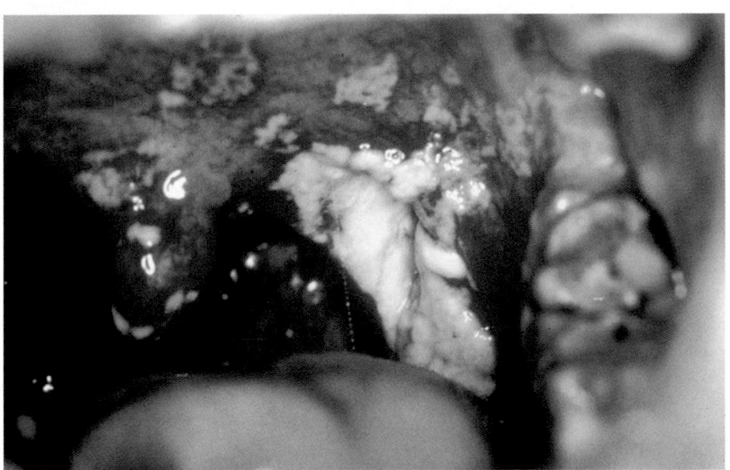

FIGURE 20.1. Oral candidiasis

(6) The "shared-care" approach with general practitioners involved in clinical management along with the hospital team is a useful model to adopt. A multidisciplinary team is often required with hospital doctors, GPs, social workers, counselors, dietitians, drug-workers, and district nurses working closely together. Most teams also have a designated "HIV liaison nurse" who plays a key role in coordinating care and oversees the smooth transition between hospital and the community.

Management of complications of HIV infection are summarized in Table 20.2.

Table 20.2. Complications of HIV infection.

Symptoms	Common cause	Common treatment
Sore mouth ± dysphagia	*Candida* (Figure 20.1)	Nystatin pastilles or suspension; amphotericin lozenges; fluconazole; itraconazole
	Herpes simplex	Aciclovir; famciclovir; valaciclovir

(Continued)

TABLE 20.2. (Continued)

Diarrhea ± weight loss	Cryptosporidium Microsporidiosis	Codeine phosphate; loperamide; paromomycin
	HIV enteropathy	Codeine phosphate; Loperamide
Headache	Cryptococcal meningitis	Amphotericin ± flucytosine; fluconazole
	Toxoplasmosis	Pyrimethamine + sulphadiazine/ clindamycin
	Lymphoma	Prognosis very poor
Cough ± breathlessness	Pneumocystis carinii	Co-trimoxazole; pentamidine
	Bacterial pneumonia	Conventional therapy
	Tuberculosis	Conventional therapy
Loss of vision	Cytomegalovirus retinitis	Ganciclovir; foscarnet
Fever/weight loss	*Mycobacterium avium* complex	Combination therapy, e.g. rifabutin, clofazimine, clarithromycin, ciprofloxacin
	Cytomegalovirus	Ganciclovir, foscarnet
	Non-Hodgkin's Lymphoma	Chemotherapy, e.g. CHOP

Other problems	Common treatment
Thrombocytopenia	Zidovudine; prednisolone (treatment often not required)
Kaposi's sarcoma (Figure 20.2)	Radiotherapy; vinblastine + bleomycin; liposomal doxorubicin; "skin camouflage"
Herpes	Aciclovir; famciclovir; valaciclovir
Genital warts	Cryotherapy; podophyllotoxin; imiquimod
Mollusum contagiosum	Cryotherapy
Seborrheic dermatitis	Antifungal (hydrocortisone cream).

(CHOP: cyclophosphamide, hydroxydaunorubicin, vincristine, and prednisolone)

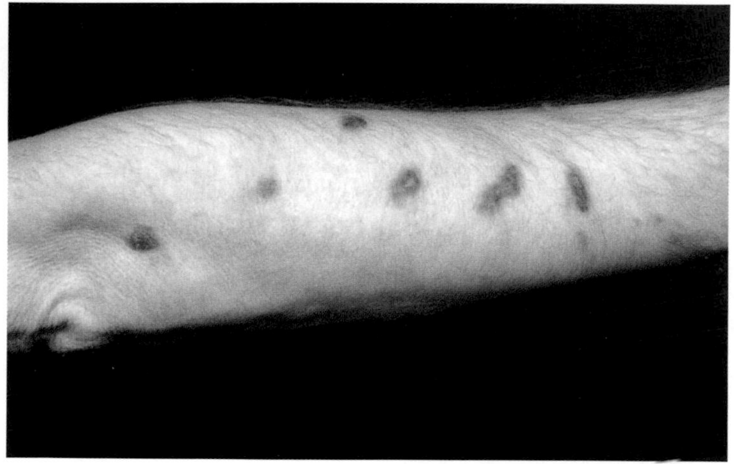

FIGURE 20.2. Kaposi's sarcoma

Chapter 21
Genital Problems in Children

Pediatrics is usually the most appropriate first line of referral for children with genital problems requiring a specialist opinion. Referral on to gynecology, urology, dermatology or GU medicine for a combined assessment can then take place if considered necessary. Consider seeking advice at an early stage, particularly if there is the slightest concern about sexual abuse. A telephone call and discussion prior to referral is often appreciated in the less straightforward cases.

21.1 GIRLS

21.1.1 Vaginal Discharge

Prepubertal girls do occasionally produce a small amount of clear, non-malodorous vaginal discharge. In addition, a slightly thicker, off-white discharge is often seen during the first week after birth and during the months preceding the menarche. A discharge which is particularly heavy or malodorous suggests an infective or pathological cause. This may be associated with vulval irritation and possibly evidence of vulval and vaginal erythema.

The more common causes of pathological discharge include the following:

(1) Infection
   (a) *Candidiasis.* Candida is an uncommon pathogen in prepubertal girls; however, symptoms, when they occur, are identical to the adult with vulval irritation and evidence of a vulvitis. *Candida* may develop on a pre-existing skin disorder such as eczema or seborrhoeic dermatitis. It is worth inquiring whether the mother has symptoms suggestive of "thrush" as transfer of *Candida* from mother to baby may sometimes occur.
   (b) *Bacterial vaginosis.* Although usually associated with sexual activity, bacterial vaginosis has been documented

in sexually inexperienced adolescents. The condition is occasionally seen in very young children; however, the prevalence of bacterial vaginosis in this age group has not been reported.

(c) Group A and Group B streptococci

(d) Escherichia coli

(e) *Haemophilus influenzae.* Although the above three groups of organisms have been reported to cause vulvovaginitis, asymptomatic carriage may also occur. Positive bacterial culture from a vaginal swab may therefore not always signify pathogenicity. A true pathogenic role may be assumed if symptoms resolve with antibiotic treatment.

(f) *Shigella flexneri.* Has been reported but generally considered an uncommon cause of vulvovaginitis.

(g) *Chlamydia.* The prepubertal vagina is susceptible to chlamydial infection. This is in contrast to the adult where the cervix and urethra are the prime sites of infection. Prepubertal chlamydial infection should raise a strong suspicion of sexual abuse, although in the very young infection may have occurred by vertical transmission from the mother at birth. This may persist for up to 2 years after birth and possibly longer. Asymptomatic vaginal and rectal infection has been reported in as many as 15% of infants born to infected mothers. Conjunctivitis and pneumonitis are more common complications and have been reported in 50–70% of exposed infants.

(h) *Gonorrhea.* This is a sexually transmitted infection and should be considered diagnostic of sexual abuse in the majority of cases.

(2) Foreign bodies

Young girls occasionally insert small objects or pieces of toilet paper into the vagina as part of normal exploratory behavior. With time these objects may give rise to a malodorous discharge. Insertion of objects that mimic a penis suggests possible sexual abuse rather than self-stimulation.

21.1.2 Genital Irritation

21.1.2.1 Vaginal Discharge

This may cause vulval erythema and irritation secondary to persistent dampness. Alternatively, vulval symptoms may be directly attributable to the initiating infection, for example *Candida*.

21.1.2.2 Threadworms
Generally considered a cause of anal irritation, threadworms may track to the vulval area and give rise to predominantly genital symptoms. The major symptom is nocturnal perineal pruritis and examination may reveal vulval and perianal erythema.

21.1.2.3 Chemical Irritants
"Bubble-bath," scented soaps, and shampoos may cause an irritant dermatitis or a true contact dermatitis. As for adults, aqueous cream is a useful soap substitute.

21.1.2.4 Poor Hygiene
Whereas excessive washing with scented soaps may cause problems, inadequate genital bathing and poor hygiene leading to prolonged exposure to urine or feces may also predispose to irritation. Non-cotton and tight fitting underwear may aggravate symptoms.

21.1.2.5 Masturbation
Children masturbate or play with their genitalia from the time their hands can reach that far. This is considered a normal part of sexual development, although it frequently generates a degree of anxiety in the parents. Public and "excessive" masturbation may be seen in the learning disabled as part of their disability. The possibility of sexual abuse should be considered in other children, particularly if masturbation is performed in public.

21.1.2.6 Lichen Sclerosus
This condition may affect young children and, to the unwary, may be misdiagnosed as evidence of sexual abuse. The clinical features are the same as seen in the adult.

20.1.3 Boys
Balanoposthitis is not an uncommon problem in uncircumcised young boys. Symptoms are usually mild and settle with simple measures, such as bathing. Recurrent inflammation is unusual and often associated with a non-retractile foreskin or poor hygiene. At birth the prepuce adheres to the glans penis in most infants. By 6 months 15% of infants have a retractile foreskin and by the age of 5 years just over 90% of boys can fully retract the foreskin. This increases to 99% by the age of 17 years. An inability to retract the foreskin may be due to phimosis which

is a pathological scarring of the foreskin, often secondary to lichen sclerosus (balanitis xerotica obliterans). Phimosis should be distinguished from a normal but non-retractile foreskin. Preputial adhesions represent a stage in the normal process of separation of the two epithelial surfaces of the glans and the prepuce and will usually spontaneously resolve without treatment.

Chapter 22
Psychosexual Problems

The limited consultation time available in the primary care setting makes it difficult to assess and advise on psychosexual problems, at least at the initial consultation. Psychosexual problems are common, may be transient, only arising within certain relationships or at certain times in life and may not be amenable to a "quick fix." Adequate time is needed to ascertain the exact problem, explore underlying tensions or issues, and develop a treatment strategy, which many primary care practitioners will consider beyond their area of expertise. Nevertheless, a great deal may be achieved during a slightly extended consultation repeated over a few sessions. Managing psychosexual problems provides the practitioner with confidence in taking a sexual history and dealing with other genital medical problems. As with other problems in primary care, specialist advice can be sought for difficult problems not responding to initial therapy.

Specialist texts are to be recommended for those dealing with psychosexual problems on a regular basis and training programs are available for those seeking more in-depth training. What follows is a very brief introduction to the kinds of approach that can be tried for the common psychosexual problems in the "time restricted" primary care consultation.

22.1 WOMEN

22.1.1 Vaginismus

Spasm of the vaginal muscles on attempted penetration is not an uncommon problem. However, before diagnosing vaginismus as a cause of painful sexual intercourse ensure there is no vulval pathology. Probably the two most commonly missed diagnoses are vulvar vestibulitis (the areas of introital erythema and tenderness may be tiny and easily missed with naked eye examination) and posterior fourchette tears. With the latter condition, there is often acute pain during sex and pain with penetration on further attempts at intercourse, until the tear heals (see Chapter 8, Figure 8.9). Vaginal muscle spasm may certainly arise secondary to these or other vulval conditions causing painful sex (e.g. vulval dermatoses, infections producing a vulvo-vaginitis) or, alternatively, may be present from the first time intercourse is attempted (primary vaginismus).

So check to see whether this is a primary problem or whether sex has previously been pain free. If the latter, ensure there is no vulval pathology.

Some women experience vaginismus as part of a more extensive sexual disorder associated with loss of sexual interest and sometimes aversion to sexual contact. This moves into the territory of requiring more intensive assessment and counseling.

Vaginismus may be encountered by the practitioner when performing a vaginal examination either by finger or speculum insertion. Inability to pass a speculum is much less common than a difficulty in opening the speculum to visualize the cervix. A question about past difficulties with sexual intercourse may unearth a long-standing problem and provide an opportunity to offer help.

22.1.1.1 Treatment

Explain that vaginismus means tightening or spasm of the muscles at the opening to the vagina (pubococcygeus) and that the objective of treatment is to help relax these muscles. As the tightening is like a reflex muscle spasm, this retraining may take a while to achieve. The muscles involved are the ones used to stop urine flow suddenly and the patient should try tensing and relaxing these muscles for 30 seconds or more a few times a day, whenever there is a convenient moment. The next step is to tense and relax these muscles whilst placing a finger gently into the vagina. Vaginal "dilators" or "trainers" are available for women who prefer not to use a finger. Start with a small size and slowly work up. Once a finger can be accommodated she should try two fingers (or a larger trainer), again relaxing and tensing the muscles. Women with vaginismus secondary to vulvar vestibulitis may find the use of lignocaine gel helpful. This can be applied after a few minutes of non-anesthetized exercises and the program repeated after the gel has had time to take effect (20-30 minutes). There should now be less discomfort and provide some encouragement. The move from finger insertion to erect penis insertion is a major step and should not be rushed. Advise partner finger insertion before penis insertion and suggest vaginal containment with the female superior or lateral position (provides the woman with more control) before starting gentle pelvic movement. Good communication between partners is essential throughout and explain that it should be a "slowly-slowly" approach, gradually moving toward full penile penetration over a period of weeks with some setbacks to be expected.

22.1.2 Impaired Sexual Desire

Try to ascertain whether this is a new problem or an occasional or persistent feeling. Is the current relationship new or long-standing and is there any discord? Is there sexual interest toward other men and does the patient have sexual thoughts or fantasies? This gives some feel to whether the problem is partner related or a more complete lack of sexual desire.

Sexual desire may be impaired by a number of factors. These include unhappiness or discord in the relationship (a common precipitant and maintaining factor for many sexual problems), partner or self-infidelity, partner's sexual dysfunction (e.g. premature ejaculation), depression, post childbirth (may be multifactorial), ill health, and ageing. Unearthing and discussing these issue may have a good therapeutic effect and further counseling can be arranged as necessary.

22.1.3 Problems with Orgasm

This may be a total inability to achieve orgasm or a situational problem with orgasm occurring under certain circumstances, such as masturbation. Sometimes expectations are high; an inability to achieve multiple orgasms should not be considered abnormal. You may have to describe an orgasm as occasionally there can be uncertainty on the patient's part as to whether orgasm has ever been reached. A reasonable clinical description would be increasing arousal, a feeling of tension reaching a climax and then being released, accompanied by a feeling of relaxation. This may or may not be accompanied by a feeling of muscle contraction.

22.1.3.1 Treatment

Check through the list of possible precipitating factors mentioned in the section "Impaired sexual desire" and address these as necessary. Make sure that foreplay is appropriate in nature and duration; this may require an overview on anatomy with reference to the position of the clitoris.

A "masturbation training programme" can achieve good results. Advise genital self-examination with reassurance that it is perfectly acceptable to touch the genitals. Some women are hesitant to do this and may consider their genitals unattractive. Reassurance and encouragement may be required. Once she is comfortable with touching the labia and the opening to the vagina she should proceed to gently touch the clitoris and the vaginal opening, perhaps contracting the vaginal muscles as she does this. The next step is to advise gentle clitoral stimulation with a finger whilst at the same time imaging a sexual fantasy. A vibrator may be used if an orgasm is not achieved after a few weeks of finger stimulation. This should be considered a temporary aid which will be required less and less as progress is made. Once self-masturbation induced orgasm has been achieved, suggest that the partner, or herself, performs clitoral stimulation during vaginal containment and then with pelvic thrusting.

22.2 MEN

22.2.1 Erectile Dysfunction

This is a common problem that may range from total erectile failure to situational or intermittent failure. The latter is unlikely to be due to a physical disorder and possible precipitating factors such as stress, depression, "performance anxiety," alcohol excess and medication side effect should be addressed. Oral medications taken before anticipated intercourse are highly effective at producing an erection and, as a consequence of this, improving confidence. Patients with total erectile failure or a history of only partial erections should be investigated for physical causes.

22.2.2 Premature Ejaculation

Rapid ejaculation is common in young men particularly when entering new sexual relationships. Ejaculation prior to or on vaginal insertion is obviously premature; however, whether the timing of ejaculation is too rapid once thrusting has begun really depends upon whether intercourse is satisfactory to both partners. Premature ejaculation can occur at times of stress and when the frequency of intercourse has been reduced, such as when a partner has been absent for some while. Detecting frustration in the partner can lead to loss of confidence and may produce even more rapid ejaculation or erectile dysfunction. In turn the partner may develop organic dysfunction and loss of sexual desire.

22.2.2.1 Treatment

The "stop–start" technique involves the partner stroking the penis to the level of arousal and then stopping before the stage of inevitable ejaculation. This should be repeated a few times before allowing the stroking to achieve ejaculation.

The "squeeze technique" involves the partner squeezing just below the glans penis at the man's indication that he has reached a level of high arousal (as with the "stop–start" technique). This is repeated a few times before allowing ejaculation.

Once the man has achieved a degree of control, the couple should move onto vaginal containment, with the partner lifting herself off at the stage of high arousal. Movement is introduced gradually once some control has been achieved.

Failures from time to time are to be expected and success may require some weeks or months of practice. It is important that the man continues to stimulate his partner sufficiently during or after these exercises.

Selective serotonin reuptake inhibitors (e.g. paroxetine, sertraline) have proved successful in treating some cases of premature ejaculation, although this is currently an unlicensed use of these medications in the UK.

22.2.3 Retarded Ejaculation

Ascertain whether this is partial failure with ejaculation occurring during masturbation or sleep or total failure. Men with retrograde ejaculation reach orgasm but fail to produce an ejaculate.

The use of a lotion as the partner stimulates the penis may enhance sensation and increase arousal. If this fails to achieve ejaculation, in future sessions the man should masturbate with the partner stroking the penis progressively earlier during the session until she can bring him to ejaculation. When ejaculation has been achieved, further sessions should focus on masturbation close to the vaginal entrance with penile insertion at the point of high arousal in conjunction with vigorous thrusting.

Just a final note on "sensate focus" treatment. This is considered an important and useful part of the management of psychosexual problems by many practitioners and is probably best left to those with expertise in this area. However, success may certainly be achieved without this approach.

Further Reading

Holmes KK, Sparling PF, Mardh P-A *et al.* (eds). (1999). Sexually Transmitted Diseases. McGraw-Hill, New York.

McMillan A, Young H, Ogilvie MM, Scott GR (eds). (2002) Clinical Practice in Sexually Transmissible Infections. Saunders.

Ridley CM (ed.) (1988). *The Vulva*. Churchill Livingstone, London.

Ridley CM, Oriel JD, Robinson AJ (eds) (1992). *A Colour Atlas of Diseases of the Vulva*. Chapman and Hall Medical, London.

Singer A, Monaghan JM (1994). *Lower Genital Tract Precancer*. Blackwell Scientific Publications, Oxford.

Adler MW (ed.) (2001). *ABC of AIDS*. British Medical Journal Publications, London.

Bunker C. *Male Genital Skin Disease*. Elsevier Saunders, London 2004.

Index

Locators in *italics* refer to figures

WMD070307

Printed in Singapore